'Knowledge of infectious diseases teaches men that they are brothers and that they stand in solidarity'.

Charles Nicolle
(21 September 1866 – 28 February 1936)
Awarded the Nobel Prize for Physiology or Medicine in 1928

'This book is a very necessary document, which sheds light on the issues of Lyme disease that are affecting patients worldwide.'

Professor Jack Lambert,
Infectious Disease Specialist, Dublin, Ireland

Dedications

To Claude Capelier, philosopher and writer, who has encouraged me during the writing of this book and who, with great foresight and intelligence, has helped me with the writing and editing.

To my family, my wife Véronique and my four daughters, Lætitia, Lorraine, Aurore and Natacha, who have always supported me with all their love, even if it was difficult for them to see my passion for my friend Borrelia *take all of my attention and time during all these years.*

To the patient groups in Ireland for supporting the work of translating this book into English.

To the European Lyme Resource Centre, an educational centre established in Dublin, Ireland, which will serve as a support for patients and healthcare providers alike (www.lymeresourcecentre.ie).

To Professor Jack Lambert, founder of the European Lyme Resource Centre, located in Dublin, Ireland, who enabled the translation of this book. Jack Lambert wrote the foreword for this book and an up-date of the situation in Great Britain and Ireland.

To the translators, Gordana Avramovic and Dr Georges S Kaye.

CRYPTO-INFECTIONS

Denial, censorship and suppression – the truth about what lies behind chronic disease

DR CHRISTIAN PERRONNE

Translated by
Gordana Avramovic, MA Linguistics, BSc

Preamble and Chapter 5 translated by
Dr Georges S Kaye

With a Foreword by Dr Jack Lambert

BOOKS

Hammersmith Health Books
London, UK

First published in French in 2017 as *La Verite sur la Maladie de Lyme* by Editions Odile Jacob, France
First published in English in 2021 by Hammersmith Health Books
– an imprint of Hammersmith Books Limited
4/4A Bloomsbury Square, London WC1A 2RP, UK
www.hammersmithbooks.co.uk

The information contained in this book is for educational purposes only. It is the result of the study and the experience of the author. Whilst the information and advice offered are believed to be true and accurate at the time of going to press, neither the author nor the publisher can accept any legal responsibility or liability for any errors or omissions that may have been made or for any adverse effects which may occur as a result of following the recommendations given herein. Always consult a qualified medical practitioner if you have any concerns regarding your health.

British Library Cataloguing in Publication Data: A CIP record of this book is available from the British Library.

Print ISBN: 978-1-78161-178-4
Ebook ISBN: 978-1-78161-179-1

Commissioning editor: Georgina Bentliff
Copyeditor: Carolyn White
Typeset by: Evolution Design & Digital Ltd
Cover design by: Madeline Meckiffe
Indexed by: Dr Laurence Errington
Production: Helen Whitehorn, Path Projects Ltd
Printed and bound by: TJ Books Ltd, Cornwall, UK

Contents

A translator's note

The embrace of intelligence is proffered with two arms: that of curiosity and that of scepticism. Within such latitude one would expect a good man, bearing sound ideas and displaying the patience of Job, to succeed. Not a bit of it! The history of medicine, of science, and generally of thought and human endeavour, is replete with tales where good turns or good deeds or good ideas 'do not go unpunished'.

The physician William Harvey in the early seventeenth century paid the price. In an epoch-making tome, Harvey fulsomely described the proper operation of the circulation of blood around the body, the first to counter 1500 years of orthodoxy dating back to Aristotle. The philosopher Bacon fired Harvey in punishment for heresy: Harvey had dared to question the masters of medicine.

Semmelweis in the mid-nineteenth century fared worse: he died in misery, having lost his wits and health long after he lost all else. It was several decades before the proof Semmelweis gave the world was accepted, that puerperal fever, the killer of millions of women in childbirth through the ages, proceeded from the accoucheur's hands being infected by the common Streptococcus bacterium – several decades, during the span of which many more women died who might have survived. The pity of it. The shame of it.

Even before fully entering Professor Perronne's narrative, whilst merely gliding over it, the similarity between Semmelweis's world and struggle, and our own – terrifyingly closer to us than Semmelweis's – leaves one incredulous. From contemporary colleagues and scientists, we had expected better. With greater force yet, we do and shall expect better. Again and again Semmelweis analysed the evidence and demonstrated his thesis, beyond the criminal threshold of proof; again and again the chorus of Polly-Burgdorfer-Scrimenti echoed this struggle trying to prove the truth about Lyme disease.

We take heed, and hail Professor Perronne's narrative. We thank him for his part and role in persisting and explaining the truth. We applaud his candour and clamour, and, through the professor's work, we celebrate the many who refused to be gagged or constrained on the long road to seeking answers.

Dr Georges S Kaye, internal medicine specialist
London, UK

Preface

A global scandal, one of the most astounding in the history of medicine, is now attracting the attention of media and public to Lyme disease and other hidden or 'crypto' infections. The primary cause of Lyme is known: a bacterium transmitted by ticks. There are effective treatments to fight it. Yet for years, health authorities and a large section of the medical community colluded (and widely continue to collude) in refusing to recognise the reality of this chronic infection and the sequelae which are often life-threatening. As a consequence of this neglect, a great number of people who are suffering tremendous pain and unimaginable distress have languished in diagnostic limbo for years. More often than not, these patients have been labelled as fabricators, hypochondriacs or plain lunatics. Millions of patients worldwide, gripped by symptoms caused by hidden, chronic infections, end up in psychiatric care or are condemned to endure stultifying and ineffectual treatments, or inappropriate surgical interventions.

Such a tragedy invites us to reflect upon the victims abandoned to terrible suffering and surreal courses of treatment, but it must also make us recognise the courage and determination of those doctors and scientists who identified the disease, who have explored its causes, and who have developed effective treatment strategies. Beyond this it behoves us to confront a crucial question: why is there such collective dissembling, or at least neglect, on the part of experts and governments alike and how can we attempt to put an end to this injustice?

Answers to such questions open up prospects of unexpected depth and richness. Whilst it would be absurd to posit a conspiracy of ill-will on the part of authorities worldwide, and specifically in America, it is nevertheless important to analyse this narrative, and seek accountability on the part of the institutions that steer, evaluate and control medical research and therapeutic trials. This is no trivial task. To such institutions and procedures falls the awesome responsibility of acting as guarantors – our guarantors – of scientific objectivity, probity and rigour. In the case of the Lyme episode, rigour turned into rigidity, and procedures morphed into dogma, to the point of thrusting us into blindness. The case of Lyme disease demands fresh perspectives and, to say the least, minds less closed and insights less constricted. In short and in Bachelard's analysis: 'Beware lest scientific tools turn into impediments – epistemological obstacles'!

How do we achieve a deeper understanding of such processes without forfeiting the benefits of the current system's framework? A reflection on this subject is an opportunity better to define the characteristics of a group of imperfectly understood maladies, caused, as is Lyme disease, by hidden infections, for which I here propose the designation of 'crypto-infections'.

Christian Perronne

Acknowledgements

On behalf of **countless patients**, I would like to warmly thank all the sufferers in France and around the world who are leading the fight for the recognition of chronic Lyme disease and related diseases – patients whose daily courage commands respect and admiration in the face of a mountain of denial and rejection. Many are enduring a terrible fight, without help.

Then I would like to thank **the few doctors in my hospital department** who have believed me and helped in the care of the sick.

I would also like to thank the **nurses, nurses' aides, and secretaries of the department** who did not fully understand this complex disease, or these patients who were so difficult to understand and treat, but who trusted me, especially after seeing some spectacular results in severely disabled patients.

Other doctors I would like to thank are:

- The courageous general practitioners, in particular those of the Chronimed group, who, under threat from France's Department of Social Security, treated and saved tens of thousands of patients, often in distress.
- Professor Luc Montagnier, Nobel Prize winner in physiology or medicine, for his support for the cause of Lyme disease and associated diseases.
- Dr Philippe Bottero, a courageous pioneer condemned for having saved thousands of sick people.
- The doctors in the Department of Social Security and in the

Order of Physicians, still a minority and obliged to remain discreet, but who show me their increasing solidarity.

I would also like to thank these **patient support associations**

- The first patient support associations: the Tiquatac.org site, the Nymphéas, SOS-Lyme and Lyme Éthique, true pioneers who, without any means, cleared the ground and made certain political figures aware of the problem.
- The first major association, France Lyme, which provided a national dimension to the debate.
- Other associations like Lympact, Lyme Sans Frontières (Lyme Without Borders), the Relais de Lyme, le Droit de Guérir, Orne Lyme, Vaincre Lyme, Lyme Team.
- Judith Albertat, former president of Lyme Without Borders, who gave a new impetus to the fight during her presidency.
- The French Federation Against Tick-borne Diseases, bringing together patient representatives (France Lyme, Lympact and Le Relais de Lyme) with a scientific council composed of doctors and researchers. Its slogan 'patients, doctors, researchers together' is a superb model for advancing the cause of patients with serenity and on a scientific basis.

My thanks too to **the leaders and numerous volunteers** of the French Federation Against Tick-Borne Disease (FFMVT) who, while fighting against their fatigue, their pains and their handicaps, joined me to carry out remarkable work, in particular to help others in distress.

I am indebted to the **scientific journals, journalists and the media**, in particular the medical and scientific journals and journalists who have had the courage to publish works diverging from the imposed 'dogmas':

- Chantal Perrin, journalist, who produced the first major report on the disease and the associated scandal for France

5 television. The report was a huge national and global success and paved the way for media debate. Chantal later wrote a remarkable book on the subject with Roger Lenglet.

- Gwendoline dos Santos of the newspaper *Le Point*, who, through her talent, inaugurated a series of spectacularly successful media events, triggering an epidemic of downloads. This public enthusiasm for the Lyme cause was confirmed by the enormous impact of several reports by other journalists on different television channels and in several newspapers.
- Isabelle Léouffre from *Paris Match* who was able to highlight the poignant testimony of patients.
- Emmanuelle Anizon from *L'Obs*, who, aware of the scale of the problem, mobilised herself and produced a major report that made it possible, through its fallout, to publicise the Lyme disease problem throughout France, with a relay in all national newspapers.
- The many doctors who signed a petition published in *L'Obs*.
- The courageous sick, more and more numerous, who agreed to come out of the shadows to testify to the media.

I must also thank the **political figures** who gradually saw the immense repercussions on the health of their fellow citizens and who joined the fight.

My thanks too to the **patients, doctors and researchers from all over Europe but also from other continents with whom I am in regular contact.**:

- Professor Michel Franck, from the veterinary school in Lyon who developed research projects on PCRs.
- Jenna Luché-Thayer for her extraordinary global combat in the defence of human rights. Her commitment at the head of a global coalition is very powerful.
- Professor Jack Lambert from Dublin, for his intelligence,

his commitment, his desire to work with me and other university colleagues to develop scientific research, education and communication in Europe. Thanks to Jack Lambert and his financial help, this English version of my book exists.

- Dr Georges Kaye, specialist in internal medicine in London, who speaks perfect French and English. Georges Kaye called me a few weeks after the publication of my book in 2017 to tell me that he read it with enthusiasm. He came to see me in Paris and started the translation of my book. We remain friends.
- Gordana Avramovic, research project manager at the University College of Dublin, Ireland, who is working with Jack Lambert, and accomplished a feat by translating the main part of this book in a short period of time.
- My wife, Dr Véronique Perronne, specialist in internal medicine and in infectious and tropical diseases, who joined me in 2018 in my department to help me in the management of chronic Lyme disease and other crypto-infections. Cheerful thanks for her huge help and support.

My thanks too to the **French but also English, Swedish, Finnish, Polish and Australian doctors** whom I helped in their defence during the violent attacks against them by the health authorities of their countries.

I would also like to thank this **institutional leader who wished to help advance research**: Ms Marisol Touraine, former Minister of Health, and her advisers for having become aware of the problem and deciding to act

About the translators

Gordon Avramovic MA Linguistics, BSc is Research Project Manager at University College Dublin, Ireland.

Dr Georges S Kaye is a specialist in Internal Medicine running a private general practice in London, UK.

About the author

Christian Perronne, doctor of medicine and of science, is Professor of Infectious and Tropical Diseases at the Faculty of Medicine Paris-Île-de-France-Ouest, University of Versailles-Saint-Quentin-en-Yvelines (UVSQ), Paris-Saclay. He was Head of the Department of Medicine at the Raymond-Poincaré University Hospital in Garches (Hauts-de-Seine) of the Greater Paris University Hospitals group (Assistance Publique-Hôpitaux de Paris) from 1994 until December 2020, when he was asked to step down because of his public statements on the management of the Covid crisis.

A former graduate of the Pasteur Institute in bacteriology and virology, he was Deputy Director of the National Reference Centre for tuberculosis and mycobacteria at the Pasteur Institute in Paris until 1998. He is former President of the Collège des Universitaires de Maladies Infectieuses et Tropicales (CMIT) and co-founder and former President of the Fédération Française d'Infectiologie (FFI, French Federation of Infectiology).

He was president of the French National Immunization Technical Advisory Group (CTV) from 2001 to 2007, the committee in charge of national vaccine recommendations. At the Medicines Agency (currently National Agency for the Safety of Medicines and Health Products, ANSM), he was a member of the anti-infective treatment group from 2000 to 2006 and chaired the working group to develop national evidence-based recommendations for the proper use of antibiotics in respiratory infections.

He has been principal investigator of several National AIDS Research Agency (ANRS) clinical research trials on HIV infection and viral hepatitis. Christian Perronne was President of the Conseil Supérieur d'Hygiène Publique de France (Superior Council for Public Hygiene of France). He was Chairman of the Communicable Diseases Commission of the High Council for Public Health (HCSP) from 2007 to March 2016, which develops recommendations for public health and vaccine policy for the Ministry of Health. He was President of the National Council of Universities (CNU), Infectious and Tropical Diseases subsection from 2007 to January 2016. He was a member of the scientific committee of the Institute for Research in Microbiology and Infectious Diseases (IMMI), a thematic institute of the Institut National de la Santé et de la Recherche Médicale (INSERM, National Institute for Health and Medical Research) from 2009 to 2013.

He was a member of a research unit at the Pasteur Institute and INSERM: UMR 1181 'Biostatistics, biomathematics, pharmaco-epidemiology and infectious diseases' (Bio2PhEID lab). He was Vice-President of the European Expert Group on Immunization (Etage) at the World Health Organization until 2015. He was Vice-President of the French Federation against Tick-borne Diseases (FFMVT). He is author or co-author of over 300 referenced international scientific publications.

Foreword

This book tells of the experience of a French 'Lyme' doctor, Christian Perronne, and readers may think it is a uniquely Gallic experience. Sadly, however, it is not. Every 'Lyme' doctor worldwide has had very similar, if not identical, experiences to those of Professor Perronne. And many infectious disease doctors who treat Lyme patients find they are working in a 'vacuum' without support; they are often 'isolated' from their peers because of their 'belief' in chronic Lyme, or they cannot perform research studies because all of their research proposals are turned down. Yet they come up with the same observations and conclusions that have been deduced in France – that patients are not making up these illnesses, that there are many occult infections out there that are being missed by clinicians (crypto-infections), and these infections are the trigger for a cascade of infection, inflammation and autoimmunity. And these infections are being missed for many reasons: poor diagnostics, a lack of willingness on the part of the 'conventional' medical community to look beyond their 'comfort zone', and other agendas. While *Borrelia*, the bacterium causing Lyme disease is the prototype, it is clear there are multiple infections that are triggering these conditions; but it is hard to move forward with a plan to better understand, investigate and treat these conditions where there is so much resistance and ignorance, and where there are political dealings behind the scenes by the 'conventional' medical community to block progress.

I have been 'confronting' Lyme for the last six years in Dublin, Ireland, and have worked with the patient groups in the UK and Ireland to better understand the situation these patients are battling with. The first issue relates to testing: the 'powers that be' stand by the fact that tick-borne infections are rare, that the current testing method is accurate, that alternative testing (i.e. by private laboratories within the EU) is not accredited and the tests are not validated, and that patients with 'Lyme-like' illnesses can have any one of many conditions including 'mystery, as yet undiscovered, retroviruses', but never *Borrelia*. When I have treated patients with chronic Lyme in my public hospital, my colleagues have refused to support my longer courses of treatment as these do not follow the official 'guidelines', but these same colleagues turn around and treat other infections for longer periods of time than set out in the 'guidelines' for those infective organisms. Indeed, I have seen many of them give patients in their private practices longer courses of treatment, but they do not do it in the public hospitals.

I have identified that many patients in Ireland have other infections besides *Borrelia*, especially *Anaplasma* and *Chlamydia pneumoniae* but my microbiology 'colleagues' in the public system have banned me from testing for other tick-borne infections as being 'a waste of resources'. When I send samples for testing to the laboratory that these colleagues 'control', these samples are thrown away. I have asked for meetings with them to discuss this problem and to educate them; no response.

I was asked by Tick Talk Ireland, the patient group, to review a 'final draft' of an Irish health executive document on Lyme disease in Ireland, which stated that 'even without treatment, *Borrelia* spontaneously disappears'. When the patient group asked me to 'challenge' these statements, I did so; I was subsequently told the document was just an 'early' draft and that it was under review. This wording was eventually removed from the Irish Lyme health executive document.

I have attempted to conduct research and get approval for my Lyme research project through my hospital's research ethics committee. It took 15 months to get approval as 'one unidentified reviewer' did not approve of my 'off licence' use of antibiotics, and I had to get a letter from another infectious disease consultant to say that he agreed with me doing research on this subject. This has never, ever been required for any research ethics proposal at my hospital before, and, by the way, my most recent Covid-19 research proposal was approved in a record 15 days (not 15 months!). Why?

I then tried to set up a Lyme resource centre in Ireland, focused on educating the public, training GPs and developing research; I announced plans and set up a launch. My public hospital 'colleague' went around and recruited a cadre of consultants, and even the hospital CEO, who were misinformed about the goals of the LRC. I was banned from conducting the launch on hospital premises and had to book a hotel nearby to conduct the launch, attended by dignitaries and patient groups from Ireland and the EU. Why?

I have conducted training sessions for GPs on tick-borne infections as I have seen many patients coming in to see me with a missed Lyme diagnosis, often instead diagnosed with 'cellulitis' or 'ringworm' when it was clear they had had a tick bite or had been in a tick-suspect area and had systemic symptoms consistent with tick-borne infections. I had many patients coming down from Donegal, in the northern part of the Republic, with these unexplained symptoms, and a group of these rural people who had been chronically unwell but with negative Lyme tests, and who had been 'fobbed off' by their GPs as 'psychiatric' or making up their illnesses. I saw many of these people who had a clear history of tick-bite exposure yet whose GPs would not even entertain Lyme as a possibility and refused to even conduct a Lyme test, having already caterogised them with another 'blanket' diagnosis: fibromyalgia, chronic fatigue syndrome, functional neurological syndrome, chronic pain syndrome and others. Furthermore, in Donegal, where I found a cluster of chronically infected patients near GlenVeigh, who had these 'mystery' illnesses, and who got better with my longer course treatment, I was asked to talk on the Donegal radio station. I mentioned that I thought there were many missed diagnoses and that GPs were not adequately trained in tick-borne infections.

I have conducted studies on *Borrelia* in ticks in Donegal, and we found about 6% of ticks were positive for *Borreliae*, including the cause of relapsing fever borreliosis. Either way, these patients were sick, and I believed in the genuineness of their illnesses; I was treating them and planning a training programme for GPs in Ireland (and the UK). I had done the same for STIs (sexually transmitted infections) in Ireland and have trained over 1000 GPs and nurse specialists over the years in these infections, with good success and appreciation.

Shortly after the radio interview, I was visited by a senior member of UCD (University College Dublin) who had received a complaint from a GP who said I had 'slagged off' the GP on the radio. I had to write an apology. I also received a very nasty letter from a GP group in Donegal, saying they did not support the way I diagnosed Lyme disease nor my approach to treatment, and they would not work in partnership with me to get their patients better. This GP group had no alternative diagnosis to offer, but clearly their impression was that the patients were 'nuts' and the cause of their symptoms could not be Lyme disease or any other associated tick-borne infection. Thus, while I teach the GPs about STIs, and this is widely appreciated, when I try to teach about Lyme disease, many reject this offer. They stand by the 'mantra' of the health authorities in the UK and Ireland that discount and discredit tick-borne infections as 'rare' and often 'made up' by patients. It should, however, be noted that studies conducted by

UCD researchers have shown that ticks on animals in Ireland are carrying *Borrelia, Anaplasma* and *Babesia*.

Not all GPs have been resistant. A number in Donegal who accept that their patients have these 'mystery' illnesses and are willing to entertain the idea that there may be an underlying infection despite negative tests, have worked together with me and their patients to get them better.

What then is the current status of Lyme disease and other tick-borne infections in Ireland? And what is the thinking of infectious disease specialists here? As in France and most other countries, it is not encouraging. Early on I reviewed a number of teenagers who I thought had *Borrelia* infection. They had positive test results from private laboratories and convincing histories of tick-borne infections. I was visited by one of the IDSI (Infectious Diseases Society of Ireland) doctors, who warned me off seeing these patients, and indeed pointed out to me that one of the patients had been hospitalised with a problem that was a parental one – a sort of 'Munchausen's syndrome by proxy'. This was a scary informal meeting where I felt quite threatened, but why blame the parents?

Later, I was asked by the Irish senate (the 'upper house' of Ireland's *Oireachtas*), by their medical subcommittee, to provide an introduction to the hearing on tick-borne infections. This meeting was set up to give the Irish patient group, Tick Talk Ireland, a forum to present the difficulties they were having, including neglect and indeed abuse at the hands of many GPs and consultants in Ireland when they raised the issue of 'Lyme disease'. As requested by the chair of the Medical Committee, I was asked to provide my presentation ahead of time, which I did. I had planned to leave this meeting within 15 minutes, to go back to patients at my hospital who had booked appointments that morning. During my 10-minute introductory statement, members of the Department of Health and about 10 consultants from IDSI, arrived at the hearing and walked in 'en masse'. Were they there to support the patient groups? Following my introduction, I was then asked by the Medical Committee to respond to a signed petition from all members of IDSI (except one, me!), which gave a 'narrative' on Lyme disease. It basically said they supported the Swiss consensus guidelines of 2016 that stated there was 'no such thing as chronic Lyme' and that a short course of treatment cured most people. As I had never seen this IDSI petition (I was somehow omitted although I am on their mailing list as an IDSI member), I was really unable to discuss the Swiss guidelines as I had been denied the courtesy of receiving the document ahead of the meeting though I had provided my document ahead of time.

(Following the meeting, I reviewed the Swiss guidelines. They refer back to IDSA 2008 communications that fail to recognise chronic, persistent infection. The IDSI petition, put together by my 'colleagues', failed to include most of the new data on persistent infection that I had provided in my presentation.)

I finally escaped from the meeting and left to go back to my patients, an hour later than planned. I later heard the 'Spanish Inquisition' against Tick Talk Ireland continued for a few more hours, all recorded on Irish TV and later distributed on YouTube. An Irish political champion, Mark McSherry, later told me, 'We were ambushed'.

I lost a lot of sleep over this event, having been 'stabbed in the back' by my 'colleagues'. And indeed they had done the same to the patient groups. Why would members of the Irish Department of Health and the medical consultants of Ireland show up in such force? I thought, as public servants, we were there to support our taxpayers and especially our sick ones, and help them to get better. I guess not.

I have applied for research grants through the EU to study tick-borne infections, most recently for an ERC grant for 'high risk', new innovations. I have previously received $1.2 million funding for HIV at the National Institutes of Health, and c.€2.4

million from the Third Health Programme EU for hepatitis C. My application to better understand tick-borne infections and chronic infection was strongly supported by three of the reviewers, but one reviewer scored me so low that my grant became 'non-competitive', disqualifying me from re-applying to the EU for this project the following year. This reviewer's comments, which were very personal in nature, included the following: 'The PI appears to be a follower of the movement 'Lyme-literate physicians' and International Lyme and Associated Disease Society' that identifies 'chronic Lyme' in many more individuals than would be justified by the responsible and rational application of consensus guidelines for the diagnosis and management of this and related infections. The PI is entitled to his opinions and the promulgation of these as he sees fit, but for scientific proposals of merit such conjecture should be backed up by empirical evidence and a more vigorous research plan.'

Consequently, I can well understand Dr Perronne's experiences with being 'ostracised' within France, with patient groups not being supported and with many patients being ridiculed. (The doctors in Ireland say this never happens but the patient groups here have put together a list of comments made, and they are not kind.) And all Lyme-treating clinicians, not just in France but worldwide, are in a fight for better understanding of these mystery illnesses with no support from the wider medical community.

I have recently put together a position paper on congenital Lyme disease which has been rejected by a number of UK journals. At the same time, a journal article recently accepted by the *British Medical Journal (BMJ)* which 'summarises' current knowledge about Lyme, once again rejects the possibility of chronic Lyme infection and, when reviewing the literature provided by ILADS (the International Lyme and Associated Diseases Society), states that the authors do not accept the 'evidence-based' publication provided by ILADS though this brings together all of the updated literature on Lyme infection. Instead, the *BMJ* review regurgitates the IDSA publication from 2008, re-regurgitated in the Swiss guidelines in 2016, and now re-re-regurgitated in 2020 and accepted by the *BMJ*. Who are the reviewers that accepted this publication? Maybe the same ones who are on the EU ERC committees? It is clearly a closed shop.

So what keeps Dr Perronne and myself and other 'Lyme-literate physicians' going? We clearly do not enjoy these attacks and ambushes and behind the scenes 'character assassinations'. The only tangible reward is that of seeing some very lovely and appreciative patients get better with these 'non-guideline' directed treatments.

To see the patients I have treated from Donegal, and from other parts of Ireland, from Scotland, Wales, England and within the EU, get better after many years of illness, has been truly rewarding. Their 'alternative' diagnoses faded away – that is, their chronic psychiatric conditions lifted; their chronic pain syndromes disappeared; their fibromyalgia vanished; their chronic fatigue syndrome evaporated. And the joy of seeing them get better, when so many other doctors had 'given up on them' because they couldn't find anything wrong, is the true reward. Therefore, the conclusion reached by multiple other GPs and specialists – that they must be making up their illnesses or they must be 'crazy' – cannot be right.

There is inspiration too in seeing a few GPs in Ireland be prepared to consider chronic crypto-infection rather than follow the mantra passed down to them by closed-minded consultants, like Chinese whispers, that: Lyme is over-diagnosed and very rare; there are no ticks in Ireland; the ticks in Ireland don't carry Lyme; tests used in Ireland are perfect; most people get better even without treatment; if you are still sick after a short course of antibiotics, then it is post-treatment Lyme disease syndrome and no further treatment is allowed; we don't accept the German diagnostic tests because they are not accredited (though the

Irish public health service ran their Covid-19 tests in these 'non-accredited' German labs' and they accepted these results). It is worth noting that the Tickplex Plus test that many patients get is a licensed test in Finland, not Germany!

Every now and then an Irish GP cops on when s/he says his/her patients get better with longer courses of treatment, and s/he supports this treatment. This is admirable and I thank them. And I thank every patient (mostly farmers and rural residents of Ireland) who have been so strong to fight for their health, and despite many negative consultations, and often negative comments from those who could not find an answer, have persevered and proactively worked to seek appropriate testing and treatment. These patients have really inspired me. The actual mechanism of why they get better will never be understood unless the EU eliminates 'negative' reviewers from their panels, and indeed negative reviewers from the medical journals, who accept nonsense and deny new science.

But for a Lyme-literate physician, it is a dangerous ocean to swim in; truly we are swimming in shark-infested waters. And throughout the UK and Ireland patients continue to be discredited and those doctors who take care of such patients are ostracised. The patients and the 'Lyme-literate' doctors know they are doing the right thing and these doctors are treating patients with the best of motives. But how do these treatments work? We don't know because the powers-that-be deny the existence of these conditions. And this fight has been going on for 30 years. Dr Perrone is not the first to fight this war, and he will not be the last. His story in France is similar to my story in Ireland, and similar to the stories of doctors in the USA, Canada, Sweden, Holland, and the UK. We all have had the same personal experiences, patient experiences, and scientific observations, often made independently. It is a tough uphill battle; IDSA is a powerful organisation, 20,000 or more strong. ILADS is made up of fewer than 1000 medical professionals with different expertise from the

IDSA doctors. It is truly a scenario of David versus Goliath. We are all rooting for David. And for Christian Perronne.

Dr Jack Lambert
Consultant in Infectious Diseases and Genitourinary Medicine at the Mater Misericordiae University Hospital and Rotunda Maternity Hospitals, with a teaching appointment at UCD School of Medicine and Medical Science; Director of the National Isolation Unit for Highly Infectious Diseases at the Mater Misericordiae University Hospital; a member of the National Viral Hemorrhagic Fever Committee of the Health Service Executive (HSE) Ireland

Introduction

To put all that follows in this book into context I would like to begin with an up-to-date set of figures regarding the current known incidence of Lyme disease in countries that are key to what follows in later chapters:

- Annual reported Lyme borreliosis in Europe has ranged from 65,000 to more than 200,000.[1,2] In 2014 and 2015, an incidence of 117 Lyme borreliosis cases per 100,000 inhabitants was found in the Alsace region of France.[3]
- In France in 2018, the incidence increased by 104 cases per 100,000 inhabitants. In 2016, the most affected region was Limousin (617 cases per 100,000), followed by Lorraine and Poitou-Charentes. Alsace was fourth (281 cases per 100,000).[4]
- In Germany, based on a retrospective analysis of health insurance data, an incidence of 261 cases per 100,000 was found for the reference years 2007 and 2008.[5]
- In the US, the incidence is still growing and the disease has spread across the 50 states. In 2016 in Connecticut, the incidence of cases was found to be 1980 per 100,000.[6]

In addition to Lyme disease due to some species of *Borrelia bacteria*, there are other pathogenic species of *Borrelia* which are never routinely looked for and other micro-organisms, mainly bacteria and parasites, which may be responsible for concurrent infections, the so-called 'co-infections'. As borreliosis and co-infections are often not apparent, hidden away within our bodies, I call them 'crypto-infections'. I'll explain more extensively the choice of this word, at the end of Chapter 1. As no tests are done routinely for most crypto-infections, there are no reliable statistics worldwide.

If we look at what happens to patients who recovered from the acute Covid-19 disease due to the new coronavirus SARS-CoV-2, we observe that some of them develop a persistent syndrome (post-Covid-19 syndrome), with fatigue, multiple pains and various disorders, a syndrome very similar to chronic Lyme disease. A hypothesis is that dormant crypto-infections with bacteria and/or parasites are awakened by the acute coronavirus infection. We'll see in this book that similar phenomena occur after other acute infections, such as infectious mononucleosis (glandular fever), infection with cytomegalo-virus, dengue or Chikungunya. These possible interactions between different kinds of infections should be better explored.

The current situation regarding tick-borne infections in Ireland and the UK

The situation in the UK and Ireland seems even worse than in France as described in detail later in the book. There is a down-play of the number of cases, virtually no recognition of chronic Lyme disease, no recognition that tests are unreliable and little understanding of the multiple tick-borne infections that a patients can be infected with from a single tick bite. In addition, there are no specialist treatment centres and in the UK not even any treatment specialists within the NHS.

Guidelines

Most UK specialists follow classic IDSA guidelines (see page 322), and in many ways are more restrictive than many other countries. The UK NICE guidelines that came out in 2018 focus only on early Lyme infection and stick by the usual mantra that Lyme is rare and easy to diagnose, that most doctors are 'skilled' in making a Lyme diagnosis, and that a short course of antibiotics will cure most individuals with 'confirmed' Lyme disease. Current guidelines are 'better' than the previous guidelines in that they allow three weeks of oral antibiotics, and then another three weeks of an alternative course of antibiotics. However, they do not provide guidance on other possible tick-borne infections that doctors should consider, and do not significantly address the issue of chronic persistent Lyme. The wording, specifically from the 2018 guidelines, to address the chronic disease state, is:

'Explain to people with ongoing symptoms following antibiotic treatment for Lyme disease that:

- continuing symptoms may not mean they still have an active infection
- symptoms of Lyme disease may take months or years to resolve even after treatment
- some symptoms may be a consequence of permanent damage from infection
- there is no test to assess for active infection and an alternative diagnosis may explain their symptoms.'

Comments from individuals in patient groups include:

'I would say that the NICE guidelines fail to acknowledge uncertainty, and base their findings on very weak and questionable scientific papers, ignoring basic science and other types of evidence. Their evidence review was very narrowly focused on clinical papers published more recently, which meant that some of the more interesting research that happened earlier and different types

> of research were not included. The final recommendations were to some extent a slight improvement on past policy and practice, for instance, it was recognised that there wasn't always a rash and that Lyme disease existed more widely than was previously advocated. However, these are only some slight changes and not enough to bring about better diagnostic practices. In particular, the guidelines around testing interpretation are extremely restrictive and fail to acknowledge the poor quality of outcomes from testing, thereby excluding a lot of patients with negative test results. This of course leads to cases being missed, and again, as suggested earlier, is circular reasoning. If you exclude people with negative test results from a Lyme diagnosis, you can argue that anything that happens after that isn't Lyme disease but something else. It's a self-perpetuating paradigm which leaves no space for individual, contextual, clinical history, and assessment for those at risk.'

The Irish guidelines discuss prevention and diagnosis of Lyme disease but do not go into detail on treatment. Most Irish consultants choose to follow the NICE guidelines or the IDSA guidelines.

Testing and numbers of cases

The numbers of cases in the UK and Ireland are hugely debated. You must get a lumbar puncture to count in Ireland, and you must have a laboratory diagnosis to count in the UK. So while Ireland says there are fewer than 20 cases annually, and 'guestimate' maybe 200 to give 'lip service' to the patient groups, there may be as many as 2500 in Ireland based on my estimates. Meanwhile, the UK records around 900 cases per year, but this number is based on strict serological (blood) testing; this does not include those with the EM (bull's eye) rash that did not get a test, and many tests are called 'false positives' where indeed they could be weak positives. Also, many with Borrelia infections never get a positive test. The current official estimate for the UK is around 2000 to 3000 new cases of Lyme disease per year. However, a study in 2019 concluded that the number is more likely to be around 8000. Without accurate diagnostic tests the debate will continue.

When patients present themselves with the results of alternative testing, not 'blessed' by the UK and Irish authorities, they are told these tests are not accredited or not validated. However, these results are often from private laboratories accredited by the International Organisation of Standardisation (ISO) within the EU. The same UK and Irish authorities sub-contract to have testing done for other infectious diseases to these same laboratories, and utilise these tests in the public hospital system to assist with diagnosis; and indeed use these test results to influence patient treatment. On the other hand, some of the UK tests which are accepted are not ISO-accredited. Thus patients are in a difficult position trying to understand the double standards involved.

GP education

While the UK and Ireland state they have education and treatment regarding Lyme in place, this mostly consists of websites with some basic information, which practitioners seldom access. In both countries, there is an attempt to downplay the extent of Lyme disease and the presence of co-infections, and there are no robust training programmes for GPs to assist them in early diagnosis and early treatment. GPs in some areas are requesting more education because they feel the NICE guidelines do not meet their needs. The Royal College of General Practitioners (RCGP) ran a one-year Spotlight project which resulted in development of an online 'Lyme Disease Toolkit' (www.rcgp.org.uk/

clinical-and-research/resources/toolkits/lyme-disease-toolkit.aspx). Training materials were developed but the project was shelved before many courses could be run.

Denigration of patients

Lyme disease is extremely politicised in the UK and Ireland and, rather than embracing new challenges to support and better understand patients, they are denigrated if they do not get better following standard treatment. If patients go to health practitioners with a history of Lyme but negative tests, they are given alternative diagnoses. In many cases these are psychiatric diagnoses, and many complain of being treated unkindly and disrespectfully by these doctors.

Access to private care

To access private care is quite difficult in UK and Ireland, and many patients travel internationally to access therapy. Only the well-off can get private appointments and private treatments, which they have to pay for themselves. No support comes from the public or private healthcare system or insurance companies in the UK or Ireland.

A number of doctors in the UK and Ireland who treat chronic Lyme and co-infections in a way that does not accord with the official 'guidelines' have been faced with Medical Council investigations. However, when the same doctors treat patients 'off licence' or extend or change treatment for other infectious diseases that do not fit the 'guidelines' they can do so without consequence. Many infectious disease doctors extend treatment for bone and soft tissue infection for periods well beyond the 'guidelines' based on their clinical assessment of the conditions, and are applauded as the patients get better. When what we call 'Lyme-literate' doctors (those who understand the condition clinically) do the same, they are criticised or even formally investigated by the Medical Council as they are not following guidelines or are prescribing 'off-licence'. The common situation is that patients get better, there are no complications from the carefully monitored treatment, and the patients have no complaints. However, complaints come from other doctors or authorities who are not patients because they disagree with 'non-guideline' based treatments that have got patients better. This does not happen for other diseases, which once again raises the question as to the motivation of the UK and Irish doctors and medical authorities.

Political activity

Patient groups have tried to work with National Health Service (NHS) bodies in the UK and the Irish Health Executive (HSE) without much success. They are rarely included as a 'token' on committees, and their concerns for the recognition of chronic infection with tick-borne infections are largely ignored.

Patients from UK and Ireland have approached governmental authorities to be their champions and advocates. Very few have had the courage or insight to support these patients in a sustainable way, and any action seems to be directly related to political rather than humanistic and medical concerns. A few shining stars include Mark Mc Sherry TD in Sligo Ireland, Alexander Burnett MSP and Donald Cameron MSP in Scotland, and Michelle Donelan MP and the Countess of Mar in England.

In the UK House of Commons, an All-Party Parliamentary Group on Lyme disease was formed but, although there was good initial interest and several meetings, interest appears to have waned and the group's website is no longer functioning. In Scotland, a parliamentary motion by Alexander Burnett MSP led to a 2017 debate in the Scottish Parliament on 'Lyme Disease: the Need to Do More'.[8] Despite demonstrating a good understanding of the issues, little more has actually been achieved since. A patient petition lodged in 2017 has taken so long to be considered by the Petitions Committee that the committee membership has almost completely changed since the first meeting was held.

In Ireland, the patient group Tick Talk called for a public hearing by the Irish Government's Medical Committee in the Irish Oierechtas. At that committee, members of the Department of Health and Infectious Disease consultants from throughout Ireland made an unexpected submission which pilloried both the patients and the clinicians treating patients outside of the guidelines. This was all recorded on YouTube. It is difficult both for patients with chronic infections and for doctors looking after such patients to experience such 'stabs in the back' and to lack support to assist patients chronically infected with these treatable infectious diseases.

Summary

In summary, the situation is bleak in the UK and Ireland. There is an unwillingness for the 'powers that be' to look at all of the scientific literature on tick-borne infections. The guidelines fail to be 'inclusive' and cherry pick the research articles they use to support their biased point of view. The UK NICE guidelines have excluded all studies of Lyme from before 2001, although many of the sentinel studies to support chronic persistent infection exist in this literature. Is this an innocent oversight on the part of Public Health of England, or an intentional omission?

An individual from one of the UK charities has summarised the situation as follows:

> *I think it's really quite astounding that an illness that clearly is increasing at an exponential rate, and that is now a risk in many different environmental physical situations, including gardens, allotments and parks, etc, should not be considered*

> *a priority for research, or policy development. I believe that the problems lie within the Department of Health, within which there is a reluctance to acknowledge any issues that need resolving and where there's a lot of scepticism about what needs to be addressed.*

Tick-borne infections are increasing worldwide, with evidence of spread in the UK and Ireland. We are taxpayers, paying for governmental health representatives and clinicians. Instead of supporting Lyme patient groups, the medical community has denied support and treatment, failed to listen to patient representatives and failed to support research. Government has failed to provide a support framework or funding to support the well established condition of chronic tick-borne infection. To deny that chronic Lyme disease occurs is to deny the right to a decent existence for UK and Irish patients, which is indeed a 'human rights' violation. Having been denied medical care and support, patients reach the conclusion that taking legal action based on being denied basic human rights is the only way forward: against the UK NHS and Irish HSE and DOH which do not recognise their plight; or against doctors who have failed to adequately diagnose and treat them.

Chapter 1

The problem of Lyme and other crypto-infections

Microbes have coexisted with human beings since the dawn of time and, for better or worse, they have contributed intimately to the organic balance, not to mention the structure and components, of our cells. However, understanding the role of microbes in the genesis of diseases is a long-term task that is far from complete. New microbes emerge regularly, such as the SARS-CoV-2, the new coronavirus responsible for the Covid-19 pandemic.

Lyme disease: a critical moment in understanding infectious processes

The microbes that cause Lyme disease have caused one of the greatest controversies in the history of medicine. Lyme disease is (usually) the consequence of an infection by the *Borrelia burgdorferi* bacterium, a small spring-like microbe that can be transmitted by various routes, but most often through the bite of a tick. The colossal number of publications devoted to it shows the intensity of debate surrounding the disease and the crucial nature of the scientific and therapeutic issues to which they relate. Lyme disease sits at the crossroads of different complementary approaches to understanding and treating infectious diseases in general. Such an understanding has never been more pressing than it is today after decades in which it was assumed infectious diseases were a problem of the past. Epidemics, and especially pandemics, occur regularly to remind humanity that they always are a problem of the present and the future. The best recent example is the emergence in 2019 in China of a new coronavirus responsible for the Covid-19 pandemic.

On the one hand, despite the large number of patients who suffer from Lyme disease in its chronic form and whose symptoms, as well as reactions to drugs, cannot be explained by another diagnosis, it curiously tends to be missed by the 'radar' of the institutions and methods put in place to ensure objectivity in the identification of diseases, their causes and their effective treatment. On the other hand, the confusing variety of disorders and symptoms that Lyme disease is capable of producing, and the diversity of therapeutic protocols in place to treat them, are difficult to explain without calling upon factors that incontestable observations have certainly highlighted, but of which we still have only an incomplete knowledge.

To begin with, the *Borreliae* family of bacteria have an ability to change form and to modulate the biochemistry of their receptors, allowing them to remain 'hidden' for many months in tissues where they are not recognised by the immune system and are inaccessible to antibiotics.

However, to keep it simple and obvious, the dissent around Lyme disease and associated pathologies seems to stem primarily from the fact that reliable diagnostic tests have never been developed. If patients find themselves bouncing from one diagnosis to another, and from one treatment to another, according to the interests of the specialists they consult, this is because the routine tests used to identify the disease too often fail to identify the responsible bacterium that is causing their symptoms.

As a result of a lack of research, at present, into many chronic inflammatory and degenerative diseases, we do not have more effective diagnostic tests than those of the Pasteur era (second half of the 19th century) to identify the possible hidden microbes involved. As far as Lyme disease is concerned, there is no lack of published scientific work denouncing the poor sensitivity of blood serum antibody tests tests, such as the Elisa and Western blot assays (see later), the only ones that doctors are authorised to use, but still there is no solution in sight, and will not be unless extensive research is funded and done rapidly.

Furthermore, to add to the confusion, clinicians in most countries including France and Great Britain are prohibited from ordering the second of these tests – the Western blot assay (which is reputed to perform better in certain countries) – if the patient has not first tested positive using an Elisa assay. This is despite our knowing from all those publications that the Elisa assay is the least reliable of the two tests. As incredible as it may seem, it appears – as I will explain later – that the Elisa test results have been deliberately calibrated so that Lyme disease remains officially a rare disease. The parameters for positive and negative have been established in healthy people (blood donors), with an *a priori* 'ceiling', requiring that the test does not identify more than 5% of patients in the general population as positive. Because of this artificial ceiling, there are many examples of patients testing negative in the Strasbourg region of France (where the incidence of Lyme disease is high), who have then tested positive in Paris (less affected by the epidemic).

Moreover, these tests have been designed specifically to detect the first bacterium identified as the cause of Lyme disease, *Borrelia burgdorferi*. Even if, as is true of recent versions of the Elisa test, they react to a few other strains of Borrelia also, these tests still remain insensitive to the large number of regional variations presented by species of this bacterial genus, of which new specimens are regularly being discovered. The lack of investment and of concern for the fate of patients is such that veterinarians now have more, and better, tests than those used for humans for the diagnosis of Lyme. This is because farmers have a direct economic interest in maintaining their livestock in good health, free from tick-borne infection.

Changes in the shape and persistence of *Borreliae* in the cells and tissues of patients, even after several months of antibiotics, have been proven in multiple studies by a number of methods (see page 128) and these strains are not being picked up by currently approved antibody tests; thus, millions of patients worldwide wander around with chronic symptoms of Lyme infection without an accurate diagnosis. It is not surprising, in those circumstances, that the symptoms they suffer from are often the subject of erroneous interpretation (as they are antibody negative) and they are often started on 'alternative treatments', as Lyme infection is discounted. Many of these alternative protocols, based on an erroneous diagnosis, prove to be ineffectual at best, and sometimes harmful to patients.

In short, we are faced with a disease with multiple and changing manifestations (see page 156) , which is poorly understood and whose pathological manifestations (symptoms and signs) can be extremely diverse.

It must be recognised that this is quite far from the usual disease archetype (i.e. a clearly identified cause, a table of easily identified clinical signs and a validated therapeutic protocol) to which the institutions responsible for monitoring medical research and practice (understandably) aspire. Nevertheless, there is sufficient evidence, together with converging data, and interpretative models based on sound knowledge, to provide a convincing explanation for the proven efficacy of some treatments for chronic forms of Lyme disease. The administration of appropriate antibiotics (which sometimes need to be changed to respond to changes in the shape and functioning of the bacteria), especially in combination with (or alternating with) other antimicrobial agents, can cure or significantly improve the condition of a large majority of patients, often previously severely disabled, and can enable them to resume a normal, active life.

Medical craze or patient insanity?

Since we now know how to successfully diagnose and treat chronic Lyme disease, why is it that a large proportion of medical research institutions and people involved in medical research in many countries, persist in denying the existence of this disease? Why do they even get to the point of abandoning patients to their illness, accusing them of fabricating their symptoms, or even demanding that doctors who try to treat them be deprived of the right to practise? What motivates them to continue to use notoriously inadequate serological tests and to sabotage research projects in this field as much as possible?

The mere fact that one is led to ask such questions illustrates the impasse that we have arrived at, and all of this in-fighting only hurts our patients. This seems so contrary – so much so that it becomes essential, at this stage, to give the reader a quick overview of the downward spiral of successive decisions, seemingly reasonable at first, which have led to this situation. I will later come back in more detail to the main episodes of this story, the conflicts surrounding the approach to Lyme disease and to 'crypto-infections' in general, with some thoughts on the way as to how to break the vicious circle, to the benefit of patients.

There is, however, no doubt that patients with Lyme disease around the world have been left high and dry by a health system more committed to defending its rituals than to helping them. This was the case in the US city of Old Lyme, which eventually gave its name to the disease. Here, a patient who had been labelled a hypochondriac by doctors, was successful in identifying and documenting an increasing number of cases similar to his own. However, the first specialist who conducted a follow-up study on this mysterious pathology believed that, as a rheumatologist, he had identified a new type of inflammatory arthritis.

According to this specialist, it was a very specific new disease that he summarily excluded from having an infectious origin, although this was suggested by other authorities. Despite his obstinacy in supporting this thesis, he finally had to renounce it when it became obvious that the bacterium responsible had been discovered. But blindness to the widespread incidence of the disease was common within health institutions.

First, as we shall see in greater detail later (page 39) and as mentioned above, the problem was compounded by the decision to calibrate blood serum test results so that the disease appeared rare, even if it meant banning other more sensitive tests on the pretext that they were too frequently positive. Then, denial about the disease was reinforced by the unsupported assertion that a relatively short course of antibiotics was enough to ensure a definitive cure; this reinforced the firm conviction that there could not possibly be any chronic forms of Lyme.

Finally, when it became clear that serious symptoms persisted for many allegedly 'cured' patients, a supposed 'post-Lyme syndrome' was invented which, although it did not explain anything and led to no effective treatment, at least allowed the medical profession to stick to the dogma. The defence of this position necessarily leads to discrediting as much as possible those colleagues who take care of patients with chronic Lyme and to denying the success, however spectacular, of certain therapeutic protocols, even if it means attributing to them an astonishing number of 'spontaneous cures'. (As an aside, 'spontaneously curing' a disease that doesn't exist is an idea that the surrealists would probably have liked: it is true that the writer and founder of Surrealism, André Breton, was trained as a doctor!)

It is easy to imagine that health policy makers, social security directors and the heads of private insurance companies, even with the best intentions in the world, are, for obvious budgetary reasons, more inclined to defend the status quo than to support the introduction of long antibiotic cures, accompanied by other antimicrobial agents and various investigations. Yet it is a short-sighted calculation, when we know that the suffering of patients deprived of appropriate care leads them inevitably to wander from medical department to medical department, where, from misdiagnosis to useless treatment, they end up, if I dare say so, costing more than if they had been cured. In these pages, we will discover the tragic stories of patients whose lives have been shattered, not only by their persistent pain, but also by the cruelty with which they have been treated by the medical and social care systems.

There is an amazing persistence in successive denials – denial of the disease, of the abundant evidence indicating its ancient nature and, especially, of the suffering of the patients; denial of the inadequacy of the current tests and of the current recommended treatments; denial of the effectiveness of therapeutic protocols used by the doctors who believe in the existence of 'crypto-infections' and treat them based on clinical suspicion and clinical response; denial of the obvious contradictions the official authorities are locked in – for example, when they forbid the most sensitive test to be used by those who test negative using a less reliable test; denial, again, of the need to develop more efficient tests that can target the diversity of strains and bacterial forms involved; and refusal, finally, to support better targeted research to validate (or invalidate) the most likely hypotheses as to the specific causes or mechanisms of the disease as well as regarding the most promising therapeutic models.

The theory of 'spontaneous generation' of disease

Nineteenth-century researchers, including Louis Pasteur in France and Robert Koch in Germany, worked in an era where the theory of 'spontaneous generation' was widespread; according to this, organisms could originate 'spontaneously' from fragments of inanimate matter. This theory, which implied that diseases could occur from nothing, or fall from the heavens, had the full support of the church, for reasons similar to those that had led it to support the idea that the Earth was flat and that it was the Sun that revolved around us: infectious disease thus appeared as a divine punishment.

These nineteenth-century scientists did, however, eventually discover the true infectious cause of many diseases by identifying the responsible microbes. These advances were made possible by developments in technology (microscopes, staining methods, culture media, animal experiments, etc). However, the theory of spontaneous generation, which we thought had once and for all been buried finds it harder to die than we had imagined and never ceases to be resurrected, in various guises that make it seem modern, especially in the dominant medical discourse concerning the many chronic inflammatory, autoimmune or degenerative diseases whose origins are still unknown. Could they be caused by 'crypto-infections? I look at this in details in Chapter 9. When the cause of a disease is unknown, it is now called 'idiopathic'. This is a word of Greek origin which sounds chic as well as learned and implies that the problem is a singular pathology the causes of which are 'particular to the proper character of the interactions that induce its appearance' – which is an elegant, obscure or hypocritical way of saying that we understand nothing about it.

This obscure term simply masks doctors' ignorance. This is the point at which the theory of spontaneous generation has arrived. Louis Pasteur was the object of jibes, and often violent attacks by eminent scientists, when he dared to assert that microbes were at the origin of many diseases. For my part, I have always taught my students that 'idiopathic' diseases are the diseases of 'idiots' (experts, not patients!) and that the infatuation with this term reflects the current ignorance about many disease mechanisms. This misunderstanding of the origin of many diseases is a breeding ground for a number of conspiracy theories, the most fashionable today being to attribute the origin of diseases to vaccines. Unfortunately, there is abundant evidence that the diseases in question existed a long time before the vaccines.

The 'planned disappearance of infectious diseases'

After the Second World War, the eradication of infectious diseases was planned at the highest political levels in many countries. They were to quickly disappear in the face of the omnipotence of Man and modern science. Advances in hygiene and nutrition, vaccination and antibiotics would quickly sweep away microbes, those intruders worthy only of the Middle Ages. The only small oversight was that our planet is full of microbes and that our very own organism contains more microbial cells than human cells. It's a tiny little detail, but life is either infectious or it does not exist at all.

The main research institutes have consequently abandoned entire areas of exploration in microbiology and infectious diseases in favour of more 'noble' sciences, such as immunology and genetics. It is clear that the mechanisms studied by the latter two fields play a major part in the processes that generate many diseases, but these would not occur without the third indisputable component, the microbes that wreak havoc by bringing foreign genetic material into the organism – our bodies.

Yet a famous follower of Pasteur, and Nobel Prize winner, Charles Nicolle, had, in the 1920s, brilliantly shown that chronic diseases could be linked to what he called *'les infections inapparentes'*, or 'silent infections', a term which was translated into English at that time as 'occult infections'. Many of the processes responsible for the development of poorly understood diseases could be due to these unseen microbes, hidden in our cells and organs: it seemed reasonable to him to expect important discoveries on this point in the relatively near future. Unfortunately, his grand vision has largely fallen into oblivion, except among a few pioneers, such as Paul Giroud of the Pasteur Institute, who had been his laboratory assistant, and the Belgian Jean-Baptiste Jadin. Jadin's daughter, Cécile Jadin is living in South Africa where she first practised surgery, before specialising in crypto-infections. Cécile recently sent me a photo of the marble plaque in front of the Pasteur Institute in Tunis where Charles Nicolle worked. It is worth noting, among other things, on the commemorative panels describing the activities of the Institute's laboratories, the wording: 'Typhus, Exanthema, Spotted Fever, Relapsing Fevers (Evolution of the Spirilla in Lice, Tick Fevers), Silent Diseases...'. Everything in this book is already prefigured there in a few words.

The microbiologist Wilhelm Burgdorfer (known as 'Willy') was of German-speaking Swiss origin, and in the early 1980s was the discoverer of the bacterium responsible for Lyme disease, to which his name *Borrelia burgdorferi* has been given. Burgdorfer knew Charles Nicolle's work very well and was a strong supporter of his theories. He had a thorough knowledge of the different species of *Borrelia* and was a supporter of the concept of silent infections. He had published work on these 'occult infections' in the 1950s. Having emigrated to the United States, he eventually became a naturalised American citizen. He was, in every respect, an exceptional researcher, owing to his powers of analysis and his extraordinary curiosity, but also to the originality of his scientific interests. This last trait was the mark of an independence of mind all the more remarkable given that, for the reasons just mentioned, the vast majority of researchers around the world had, since the Second World War, preferred to abandon the field of microbiology and infectious diseases, now considered outdated and unprofitable.

Burgdorfer was specifically a medical 'entomologist', specialising in diseases related to insects and 'creepy-crawlies'. It seems he worked for the US military and new evidence about his work has recently been published in the book *Bitten*, of which more on page 294.

Ticks, ethics, antibiotics and politics

In this tick business, ethics are being abused. As we shall see in the course of this book, there is a quite staggering denial of the diseases transmitted to humans by ticks, including but not limited to Lyme disease. Moreover, the controversy about Lyme is also coming up against the full force of the world war declared, not against microbes, but against antibiotics. Today, a 'woke' doctor must be 'anti-antibiotics' despite our knowing that, together with public health measures like sanitation, clean water, drainage, and vaccines, antibiotics are one of the main causes of the spectacular increase in the world population and the lengthening of human life. In comparison, medical resuscitation makes a much smaller contribution. 'To be pro-antibiotic or anti-antibiotic that is the question!' for our medical Hamlets, anyway. It's good to be 'anti' but against what? Against undiagnosed, untreated, abandoned patients?

This point of controversy is crucial because every doctor must be concerned about sparing existing antibiotics by avoiding their abuse or misuse, because of the risk in contributing to the increase in resistance of bacteria to these wonderful drugs. Unfortunately, the current extremist debate has caused the pharmaceutical industry to flee, and they no longer develop new antibiotics. A famous 'anti-antibiotic' advertisement was circulated within the Greater Paris University Hospitals group, Assistance Publique – Hôpitaux de Paris. We can see a doctor climbing on a tree and sawing the branch on which he is sitting. The message is clear: if he continues to prescribe too many antibiotics, he will be facing disaster. However, there is also the possibility that by consistently denigrating antibiotics and preventing their use, we will see the reappearance of certain infections that have almost disappeared and, more importantly, we will see research on this essential class of drugs dry up for a very long time. Yet thousands of researched chemical compounds with antibiotic, or more generally antimicrobial, properties are stored in the archives of pharmaceutical companies, for lack of any initiative or incentive to develop them.

Moreover, the experience of many doctors, confirmed by certain publications, for example the numerous research articles by Ying Zhang and colleagues, cited in this book, gives us good reason to believe that there are non-antibiotic products, including medicinal plants that can be effective in the maintenance phase of treatment of chronic Lyme disease and associated conditions. There are therefore possible solutions that could get us out of this head-on opposition between differing schools of thought, especially if we could one day pursue research in this field. This is perhaps a dream, because so far Lyme disease and more generally crypto-infections are the few conditions for which no serious research has been funded for 30 years. Unfortunately, if politicians and health-system leaders continue to bury their heads in the sand as they have been doing throughout the Lyme disease saga, science and the sick will suffer, and this will only exacerbate this looming pandemic health disaster.

This is all the more unfortunate because 'silent' or 'crypto' infections existed long before this denial of Lyme disease. Polemics have unfortunately created a lasting 'code of silence' stifling all research and thus blocking all progress. Basically, in its natural state, the infection is already hidden, but in addition, it is being artificially hidden – experts in charge of writing recommendations on Lyme disease are hiding a lot of information or trying to discredit those who escape their censorship.

After decades of denial, political awareness is gradually building in many countries. We must thank the courageous politicians who are working at the highest level to try to take us out of this crisis.

Health authorities do not have the right to avoid the issue by remaining above the fray and letting the debate become a quarrel between experts or learned societies that have never been interested in the problem. This is an emergency but unfortunately, the lack of reliable diagnostic tests is responsible for the absence of good statistics. In this context, it is difficult to convince politicians of the reality of this emergency. I appreciated the dedication of Mathieu Foucaut who, in his 2015 book *Lyme Disease: The Silent Epidemic. A Fight for Our Lives*, says, 'To the State, that is not saving my life', and, as the last sentence of his Preface comparing the current state of the Lyme pandemic with the initial stage of the AIDS epidemic, which was also long denied: 'Such a serious epidemic must not start again. Not in the way the sick have experienced it, that is, in the midst of incomprehension, suffering, harshness, abandonment, loneliness, rejection and cowardice. Let's never go through that again!'

The concept of 'crypto-infections' – the missing link between Pasteur and Freud

Pasteur and Freud studied unexplained diseases from radically opposing perspectives, yet their approaches are complementary in more ways than one. Pasteur, as we know, was one of the founders of microbiology – the study of organisms that cause disease – and shared with his German colleagues, Friedrich Henle and his student Robert Koch, the 'germ theory of disease'. In Freud's work, the psyche, which regulates the play of impulses and unconscious symbolism, manages an energy, one of the sources of which is biological and therefore capable of being modulated by the organic state of the subject. In other words, Freud acknowledged that a person's physical state could affect their emotional state. However, Freud was also open to the idea that one day biochemical mediators would be discovered through which psychic conflicts could lead to psychosomatic disorders or to organic diseases – in other words, that a person's emotional state could lead to physical illness as well as to symptoms with no apparent physical cause.

This opens a field for reciprocal interactions between the 'Pasteurian' infectious processes induced by microbes and the manifestations of the life of the mind. However, when it comes to chronic 'silent infections', it appears that while persistent microbes are at the root of real organic diseases, the psyche (the 'mind') can modulate the evolution of symptoms. We have proof that this is the case from time to time when a patient, apparently cured of chronic Lyme disease, relapses within two weeks following great stress.

Chronic Lyme patients find themselves, in some respects, in a no-man's land between microbiology and psychoanalysis. The microbiological tools inherited from Louis Pasteur's school have their limits and do not detect microbes hidden within our cells or tissues. On the other hand, these patients who constantly complain of symptoms without any easily identifiable objective cause of their ills are the subject of numerous psychoanalytical theories. It must be admitted that this is a huge 'market' for psychiatrists, psychoanalysts and psychologists, because most of the patients' complaints are subjective – that is to say, not proven by a doctor's examination or tests. When the doctor does not understand anything about what is happening to a patient, it is a well-known fact that it must all be in the patient's mind. It is difficult, in the medical sphere, to escape from the idea that it is all equivalent:

subjective complaints = 'functional' pathology
= hysteria or hypochondria

Throughout the world, millions of people suffering from chronic diseases are consequently looked after by psychiatrists.

Recently, a well-known professor of psychiatry at a major university hospital in Paris called me to tell me of his distress: his fellow general physicians and rheumatologists at the hospital spent their time sending him 'madmen' who said they had Lyme disease. He was outraged because, for him, all these patients were not crazy at all, but did have an organic problem that he could not explain himself. I congratulated him on his approach, adding, in a joking tone, that we could also congratulate ourselves that he was not a 'crazy psychiatrist'. I note that more and more psychiatrists have recently begun to react in this way, which is excellent news for the sick.

Diagnostic difficulties affect diseases other than Lyme. Indeed, many 'idiopathic' diseases may have an unknown infectious cause. At present, however, the 'star' disease for those protesting against the system is Lyme disease, because of its frequency and extent. Its 'media success' is such that, in the absence of conclusive scientific data, some would like to blame all the miseries of the world on this disease.

Like Dr Cécile Jadin who I mentioned before, I think it would be preferable to abandon the name 'Lyme disease', which focuses our attention on a single type of bacterium – the one first identified in patients in the city of Old Lyme in the United States: *Borrelia burgdorferi*. It's the tree that hides the forest. We should speak of 'borrelioses' to take into account the multiple species of *Borreliae* that cause chronic diseases in humans, and, of course, to research the countless co-infections, such as *Bartonella, Rickettsia*, or *Babesia* already known or to be discovered in the future. Scientific publications show that many inflammatory or degenerative processes can be due to other microbes (*Borrelia* species other than *Borrelia burgdorferi*, other types of bacteria, parasites, fungi, viruses – see Chapter 2). We need to be able to explore acute, subacute and chronic phenomena caused by vector-borne infections (from ticks, mosquitos and other creatures), but also infections transmitted by other routes. We must take into account active infections but also latent forms that may become active later. Many terms have been suggested: 'silent infections', 'occult infections', 'hidden infections', 'stealth infections', 'cold infections', '*syndrome post-piqûre de tique*', 'tick-associated poly-organic syndrome' (TAPOS), 'poly-organic chronic syndrome', 'multiple systemic infectious disease syndrome' (MSIDS), etc. The new official spelling in France is '*syndrome persistant polymorphe après une possible piqûre de tique*' (SPPT), which means 'persistent polymorphic syndrome possibly due to a tick bite'. More of this in the last section of the book (page 281).

Following the historical and scientific legacy of Charles Nicolle, I use the term 'crypto-infections' ('hidden infections'), which has the advantage of being short and identical in French and English, while covering a wide range of organisms and symptoms, thereby guaranteeing a broad and open approach to the topic. And that is how I will approach the topic throughout this book.

Chapter 2

The need for accurate diagnosis

Listen to what patients say

Lyme disease is at the forefront of poorly understood diseases. It often presents with a variety of subjective signs – that is, symptoms not visible to others and only experienced by the patient. Modern medicine treats primarily on the basis of the results of scans, biological examinations and/or tests rather than by listening to what patients say they are experiencing, so we end up with an 'imaginary disease' epidemic, decreed as such by the imagination of doctors alone, but which totally destroys the lives of millions of people, and with a profound impact on their families.

The French playwright Molière was taken at face value far too readily; he was seriously ill when he wrote *Le Malade Imaginaire (The Imaginary Patient or The Hypochondriac)* and, as you may know, had a haemorrhage as a complication of tuberculosis while he was playing this character in the theatre. It was during the fourth performance, at the final stage of the play. He died shortly after the curtain fell.

Molière mocked 'imaginary patients' for pretending to endure non-existent ills and pinpointed the pleasure that they felt in submitting themselves to the absurd prescriptions of doctors, who were as ignorant as they were pretentious, but skilful in exploiting their patients' delusions. In fact, he was only too aware of the pains of a real disease. At the same time, he was well placed, alas, to reveal the incompetence of doctors who knew nothing about the causes of his illness but who nevertheless offered useless treatments so as to look knowledgeable and charge a fee. I cannot but think that Molière would have thoroughly enjoyed reading about the saga of Lyme disease.

Since the beginning of my medical career, I have gradually learned to treat and even cure a considerable number of these '*malades imaginaires*', who were in great physical and psychological distress and who were probably suffering from one or more 'crypto-infections'. Medically, it has always seemed obvious to me that a patient knows his/her body and how it feels better than the doctor. What gives so many doctors the right to declare with certainty to their patients: 'The symptoms you are describing are impossible!'?

Such doctors should read *Le Petit Prince (The Little Prince)* by Saint-Exupéry and the words that the author gives to the fox: 'It is only with the heart that one can see rightly, what in essence is invisible to the eye'.

This is the right moment, I believe, to quote two short excerpts from the hundreds of letters I receive each year, chosen from among many others in the same vein: nothing is more telling or more moving than these direct testimonies. They challenge us; they force us to consider that, whatever we think about the possible causes and treatments of Lyme disease, that it would be a disgrace to let down patients who are the victims of this pathology.

Letter 1

It is not because I was taken for a madman that it is outrageous, because madmen must also be respected in their human dimension; no, it is because I was not taken for what I was that it is so offensive, thereby missing the true cause of what was eating at me for so long. One feels deprived of one's suffering, of one's history, by the influence of analytical techniques that become the only judges deciding our lives. [...] Yes, I wanted to take my own life, to escape from the stigma doctors make patients like me bear by marking us with the red-hot iron of "imaginary patient" with fantasised pains, and from the guilt which results from it. [...]

I thought of taking my life, not because I no longer loved life, did not wish to travel the Hindu Kush mountains of my Afghan friends, did not appreciate the skies scattered with cirrocumulus bursting with beauty at sunset, did not like to read Cioran, Rousseau or Dumas. No, I only wanted to take my life to *escape from my pain.*

Letter 2

Hello Professor,

I am the brother of one of your patients whom you have helped to fight Lyme disease. I want to thank you from the bottom of my heart and on behalf of our whole family for your work.

I will not talk about the remarkable work you have done on the purely medical treatment side, because although I've obviously done a lot of research, I don't claim to be able to say anything about it. For me there are two major points on which, in a purely factual manner, your success cannot be denied:

- the medical results
- the effect on morale...

Those two are undeniably related by the way.

> The medical results first of all are spectacular, because after years of descent into physical hell, my brother has lived through a real rebirth – thanks to you. Not everything is perfect obviously; with these serious diseases one never really completely recovers, but he can now live a normal life and that is the main thing when one has been so unwell. It was with great pleasure that I was able to share moments with my brother on a tennis court or during hikes in Corsica again. Thank you; that is priceless [...].
>
> My brother is also my best friend, and as such you have given me both of them back thanks to your perseverance and knowledge about this complex disease. You also gave him back to his two daughters and to his wife who had lost hope.

In other cases, the refusal to recognise the illness becomes a convenient excuse for not paying for care, at least in France where we have health insurance that may or may not reimburse a part of what patients have to spend on healthcare. Thus, it was for a farmer from the Loire region who, in what should have been his prime, was suffering from terrible muscle weakness and various neurological complications. He was summoned by a doctor from the Mutualité Sociale Agricole (MSA) (health insurance for agricultural workers here in France) who refused to give the diagnosis of Lyme disease on the grounds that his blood serum antibody test was negative and did not hesitate to mention multiple sclerosis despite the absence of confirmation of this diagnosis by neurologists at the university hospital where this patient had nevertheless been hospitalised many times. The patient was very disabled, but nobody took him seriously. His wife testified: 'He walks like a little old man. We are crossing the desert. He is clinging on to his cows, figuratively, but also literally. He finds that his condition deteriorates when he stops taking antibiotics... .'

Many patients complain of the many obstacles put in the way of their requests for care, which add to the burden of their symptoms:

Letter 3

At 45, I now live like a pensioner; my life includes a physiotherapist, a social worker, numerous administrative procedures, claims and photocopies, daily care from a home nurse, hospitalisations, medical appointments, etc. It is a full-time job! But what a long journey... I have baffled many doctors and had a huge variety of tests, for which I was criticised later. Multiple false tracks. I most definitely do not fit into any of the boxes... The pain centre at the university hospital threw me out saying: 'Madam, we can do nothing more for you; you will suffer all your life; there is nothing to be done. Goodbye'. Meanwhile, "Let us laugh a little bit whilst waiting for death," as Pierre Desproges said.

Some people can't contain their anger any longer:

Letter 4

Let the doctors who refused to treat me and who chose provocation, who ridiculed me, who chose quarrelling and ignorance, who even insulted their colleagues, with slanderous accusations and denunciations, finally realise that they have completely failed in their profession and sincerely regret it... .

Few influential patients dare to 'admit' that they have Lyme

Unfortunately, today, publicly revealing one's diagnosis of chronic Lyme disease is not yet common. While disclosure by well-known personalities of their HIV status, the virus responsible for AIDS, has become quite common, very few people cured of chronic Lyme dare to talk about it. The disease still carries a 'psychiatric' connotation and my former patients are afraid for their work/jobs, fearing that their positions of responsibility will be taken away from them. I treat a few celebrities, and one singer told me that it was out of the question for ''this to be made known', otherwise the insurance premiums for her shows would skyrocket. When, in June 2015, Avril Lavigne, the Canadian singer and songwriter, revealed to the world, bursting into tears in front of television cameras, that she was suffering from chronic Lyme disease and that she had experienced the hell of medical denial; she showed immense courage. Let us hope that this revelation has been of help to many sick people throughout the world who are facing the suspicious indifference of so many doctors. The suffering caused by Lyme disease to supermodel Bella Hadid and her mother Yolanda also made a great impression on the general public.

Lyme disease affects all social and professional groups. It is not just farmers and hikers who are affected but also many city dwellers in regular contact with nature or domestic animals. Lyme disease for a farmer who no longer has the strength to get up to plough his/her fields or look after his/her animals is a disaster not only for himself, but also for the whole farm, especially when the health insurance experts put him/her in the 'lazy impostor' category.

To physical pain, and to their family's distress in the face of dwindling farm income, are added anger, resentment and the shame of being considered a 'fake patient'. Every aspect of life is affected and seems to come together to lead the patient to despair, even suicide, which unfortunately happens regularly according to the testimonies of my patients from the countryside. Distress can also be major for some of my patients with highly responsible jobs – CEOs, graduates of the Ecole Polytechnique working in very sensitive industrial sectors, etc. Fortunately, there is often a lot of mutual support between patients, and some of those who manage to get better, even partially, find the energy to help others or at least keep them informed.

During a meeting organised by a patient support association, *France Lyme*, I met the 'godmother' of this association, Sandra Olivier, herself ill. She is a great sportswoman who has been world champion in orienteering. These competitions often take place in forests/woodland, where contestants must run with a map and a compass to find control points placed along the course. After running through the forest, she fell ill and, as she herself said in public, she suddenly went from world champion to 'vegetable'. Now she is doing a remarkable job of raising awareness amongst young people in schools and sports clubs.

Even doctors are getting sick

For some time now, I have been seeing an influx of doctors, vets and scientific researchers with chronic Lyme disease at my clinic. I'm even starting to see sick psychiatrists! One's outlook on the disease changes immediately one becomes sick oneself or someone close to one is affected. Suddenly, those doctors and scientific colleagues encounter the denial from their peers and find access to care closes everywhere. Several of them have told me: 'I will never again practise medicine the way I used to'. Let us hope these doctors and scientists make converts in their professional environments. For a while now too, I have even seen medical students and residents who are suffering from chronic Lyme and who, in turn, experience the disbelief around them.

In September 2015, I received a letter from a former colleague, now retired, whom I knew well but had not seen for years. We had worked together on the editorial board of the infectious and tropical disease textbooks for our students. This former professor of infectious and tropical diseases, and former head of department in a university hospital, wrote to me:

Letter 5

Dear friend,

I've been retired for a few years now. I admire everything you do for Lyme disease, of which I've seen a lot of cases in my department. Among other things, I have observed 'pseudo-psychiatric' manifestations that I am sure you are aware of. I have always disagreed with my colleagues at the hospital about this. [...]

Yours and good luck in your fight to make Lyme disease known... and Bravo...

All of a sudden, I felt less alone, but to be truthful, it is the only testimony that has been addressed to me in this way by a university colleague.

On the other hand, I remember another professor of infectious diseases very well, also retired, who, at the Lyme Consensus Conference in 2006, stood up like a devil in the middle of the amphitheatre and told the audience in a very firm tone that, throughout his career, he had never seen a single case of Lyme disease in his region (which is, however, full of it).

Professor Pierre Godeau, one of the greatest French internal medicine specialists and member of the National Academy of Medicine, had invited me to speak about Lyme disease in the internal medicine department of the Hôpital de la Pitié-Salpêtrière in Paris when he was already retired. He had believed in my work straightaway. Sometime later, he called me informally to ask if I would help one of his good friends, a hospital physician who was a victim of chronic Lyme disease. Such a mark of confidence on the part of this very great doctor was a huge encouragement to me.

Incorrect treatment recommendations

More and more of my hospital colleagues believe in the existence of chronic Lyme and related diseases but refuse to treat patients outside the recommendations from learned societies, even though these are totally inappropriate. Nowadays, doctors are afraid of prosecution and understandably wish, despite their beliefs, to keep their licences to practise their profession.

Erythema migrans is a red rash (often described as a 'bull's eye rash') on the skin that often appears around the spot of a tick bite and gradually widens. Reik and Burgdorfer (1986) pointed out, however, that erythema migrans occurs in fewer than 50% of cases before Lyme disease spreads.[188] According to Berger (1989), only 14% of patients who develop an erythema migrans were aware of the tick bite before the rash appeared. Physicians should be aware that, in the presence of a primary erythema migrans, a blood serum antibody testing is usually negative and therefore diagnosis should be clinical (based on signs and symptoms) at this stage. However, many practitioners still mistakenly believe that a positive blood test result is necessary for early diagnosis.

Even when doctors correctly identify the primary phase of Lyme disease and agree, usually under pressure from the patient, to prescribe an antibiotic, the dose and duration of treatment are often not appropriately prescribed, which makes these treatments ineffective in preventing the chronic progression of the disease. Each patient should be vigilant and demand that they receive the correct antibiotic treatment. The guidelines (in France), as the Haute Autorité de Santé (High

Authority for Health – HAS) reminds us, for an adult are: 3 to 4 grams per day of amoxicillin or 200 milligrams per day of doxycycline, for *at least* two weeks.

However, even in the 2016 edition of the core reference textbook written by French professors of infectious diseases, the *E. Pilly*, in the chapter on Lyme disease, written under the authority of the National Reference Centre (NRC) for Borreliosis based in Strasbourg, it is stated, without any supporting research results, that EUCALB, which was the European Concerted Action on Lyme Borreliosis, recommends giving only a single dose of 200 milligrams of doxycycline, not to be repeated, for an erythema migrans. How can such misinformation be disseminated? It is seriously problematic when we see the subsequent damage caused by a disease initially treated with a 'homeopathic' dose such as this. This guideline of a single dose of antibiotic was established in clinical studies as a preventative treatment suitable for people at risk of tick bites, but who had no current signs or symptoms of disease. Recommending this single dose to treat an erythema migrans is a serious medical mistake. All this saddens me all the more as, having been rapporteur to the Medicines Agency for the marketing authorisation (MA) of amoxicillin, I know this file particularly well.

Eric Dournon, the French pioneer in the study of Lyme disease, of whom I will speak later (page 141), must be turning in his grave; he was an ardent defender of reasonably high doses of antibiotics in the primary phase, because he had observed from the first known cases of Lyme disease in France, that too low a dose of amoxicillin was ineffective. However, and I was amazed by this, the Social Security (France's public health insurance) has, on several occasions, with patients I know, refused reimbursement for the correct treatment of erythema migrans recommended by the HAS, by intervening 'fraternally' with the patient's doctor and the pharmacist to reduce the dose and duration. It is truly disgraceful.

The three stages of Lyme disease

If untreated at the primary stage, the disease will quietly progress to its secondary form in a few weeks to a few months and then, in a few years, to its tertiary form. At each of these stages, Lyme can manifest itself as anything and everything. Like syphilis (caused by a similar bacterium) in its day, it has been described as 'the great imitator'. The only routine method available today to establish a diagnosis at these late stages is, I say again, a very poor blood serum antibody test.

This transition to chronic disease is explained by the fact that *Borrelia burgdorferi* can persist in bodily tissues even after antibiotic treatments, as animal models have shown, notably in remarkable studies conducted in the United States in monkeys, published by Monica Embers (2012; 2017). This property is not exclusive to the *Borreliae*. Indeed, dormant and persistent forms of bacteria of other types can escape antibiotics and be responsible for latent infections. Clinicians do not have a diagnostic test to check for *Borrelia* persistence. *Borrelia burgdorferi,* having a complex genetic structure, is a highly adaptable micro-organism capable of evading the immune response through various processes. This bacterium can survive both outside and inside the body's cells.

Diagnostic issue 1: Calibration of blood serum antibody tests

It is worth taking a closer look at how a small group of 'experts' imposed a particular blood test for Lyme on the whole world. The Infectious Diseases Society of America (IDSA), and the European Concerted Action on Lyme Borreliosis (EUCALB), recommend a two-tier test, the first step being an Elisa assay using the historical American *Borrelia burgdorferi* strain B31, derived from ticks and grown in vitro (in the lab). If the Elisa test is positive, the second step is confirmation by an IgG and IgM antibody Western blot. According to their recommendations, the Western blot should not be performed if the Elisa is negative, saying that it is less sensitive.

When Lyme blood testing was developed, no reliable method was available to be used as a standard. Since most of the signs and symptoms are subjective as I have said (that is, they cannot be seen or measured), or are not specific (that is, they can be seen in other diseases), no objective clinical diagnostic score could be established. Low culture yield and difficulty in using this technique were other major obstacles. As I indicated in Chapter 1, a positive threshold value for blood serum tests had to be determined arbitrarily. This arbitrary rule was decided by a small group of 'experts' and imposed on the whole world, as I have said. The threshold value for positive/negative was determined not by testing patients, but by testing blood from healthy blood donors. In the late 1970s, when Lyme disease was discovered, it was described as a rare and regional phenomenon.

Borrelia burgdorferi culture or genome detection by polymerase chain reaction (PCR) may occasionally confirm the clinical diagnosis in patients whose blood test is negative ('seronegative'), but none of these methods is, even in 2020, sensitive enough to be considered a reliable diagnostic method, especially routinely.

A test 'limited' by design

Up until 2006, I knew from numerous scientific publications in the key medical journals that Lyme blood testing was often faulty, but I had no idea of the extent of the damage and, above all, that this was intentional. I made this amazing discovery at the 2006 French Consensus Conference organised by the Société de Pathologie Infectieuse de Langue Française (SPILF), the French infectious Disease Society, to which I will return later. During this conference, Marc Assous, whom I had got to know a few years earlier as a trainee doctor in the old Claude-Bernard Hospital, gave a presentation which, unwillingly, illuminated for me one of the major problems of *Borrelia burgdorferi* blood serum testing.

Marc explained that the test was not calibrated on patients but on healthy blood donors (as I have said) and that the 'club' of self-proclaimed European 'experts', EUCALB, required all laboratories in Europe to calibrate their tests on 100 blood donors from their region, so that there would never be more than 5% of people in a given area detected as 'seropositive' for *Borrelia burgdorferi.*

EUCALB was created in Europe in 1996 on the initiative of a few experts in order to transmit the 'reliable American findings' of IDSA to all European laboratories and impose its rules. The organisation was for some time funded by the European Union. I thus discovered that a system of testing intended to maintain Lyme as a 'rare' disease was imposed by a group of experts without any scientific support. When I saw the slide and listened to Marc Assous, I couldn't believe my eyes or ears. At the end of his presentation, I asked Marc for further explanation on this point. He answered that this strategy was logical because, with any other method, 'We would have too many patients diagnosed with Lyme disease and we wouldn't know what to do with them'!

I was appalled, as you can well imagine. This immediately reminded me of the patient from Alsace, briefly mentioned in Chapter 1, who, by taking the train from Strasbourg to Paris, had been able to benefit twice, in each of these cities, from a blood serum test using the same technique and who had gone, in the course of his journey, from negative to positive. As the population of Alsace is greatly affected by *Borrelia,* the threshold of 5% is reached much more quickly than in Paris, and thus, in proportion, many more Alsatian patients are placed in the 'not sick' box.

Marc Assous published his report from the conference in 2007, in the journal *Médecine et Maladies Infectieuses,* mentioning this locking at 5% of blood samples imposed by EUCALB.[9]

I could then see why the Americans had been careful not to write this instruction in an official document. On the IDSA and EUCALB websites, it was clearly stated that blood testing is calibrated on 100 healthy blood donors, but the figure of 5% of the local population did not appear, and for good reason. If this method had been applied to HIV, it would represent a huge health scandal. For Lyme, it doesn't appear to disconcert anyone (except patients, of course), probably because the population is not aware of the problem. In fact, only acute or subacute very symptomatic cases of Lyme disease are visible, like the tip of the iceberg. Eventually, the EUCALB website disappeared in 2017, leaving no trace… .

As a result of this approach, many patients with signs and symptoms compatible with Lyme disease, but whose blood serum antibody test is negative, are left to their fate. To add insult to injury, patients with these same symptoms who, fortunately, have a positive result are often declared not to have Lyme disease, on the pretext that their test is a 'false positive'. In any blood test which, by definition, is an imperfect test requiring calibration, there may be a tiny proportion of false positives, but this is exceptional. Even if *Borrelia burgdorferi* could cross-react with other *Borrelia* species, which has never been demonstrated, the test would still be positive for borreliosis requiring treatment.

I saw poor foresters, bedridden at the age of 55, who suffered from rheumatic symptoms with major neurological and cardiac problems, being rejected by 'experts' so that their disease would not be recognised as 'occupational', even though their Lyme disease blood test was positive according to official criteria. Similarly, many patients in the chronic phase of their disease have immunoglobulin M (IgM) antibodies which, for most infections, only exist in the early phase of the disease. However, for Lyme disease, IgM antibodies can persist for months or years when the disease is evolving. As a result, 'experts' do not recognise their chronic disease, since they have these antibodies known to be typical of an initial phase.

Modern medical practice tends to pride itself on being 'evidence-based'. For this reason, most doctors rely on blood tests rather than signs and symptoms and do not admit the diagnosis of Lyme disease without serological evidence. The neurological forms of Lyme, often responsible for meningitis, encephalitis, paralysis and/or neuralgia, called 'Lyme neuroborreliosis', are often seronegative (i.e. with a negative blood serum antibody test result). Yet these manifestations of the disease, particularly acute or severe neuroborreliosis, can have disastrous consequences, including chronic neurological damage or even death. A review of the scientific literature shows that the diagnosis of Lyme neuroborreliosis is often difficult to prove. The sensitivity of measuring specific antibodies in cerebrospinal fluid, which is collected by lumbar puncture, is between 55 and 80%. In a Swedish study, antibodies were present in the serum of only 23% of children with neuroborreliosis.[34] Neurocognitive tests (measurements of memory and brain concentration problems) or brain imaging by PET-scan (positron emission tomography) can help provide objective evidence of a real disease.

Curiously (but fortunately for these patients), the experts who shamefully declare, against scientific evidence, that the Lyme blood test is perfect and detects almost all patients, do recognise nevertheless that it does not diagnose all patients, in particular, those suffering from neuroborreliosis. It is surprising to observe, with regard to Lyme, how much the 'experts', who make the law in this field, often let themselves go on to make completely contradictory statements without blinking and without having to justify themselves before the health authorities.

Thus, the European recommendations published in 2007 in the journal *Neurology*[19] under the leadership of Blanc and Jaulhac, doctors at the Strasbourg University Hospital where the National Reference Centre (NRC) for Borreliosis is located, stipulate that pragmatic diagnostic criteria, in particular the response to an empiric antibiotic treatment used as a diagnostic test, are relevant for diagnosing neuroborreliosis in cases of negative blood tests. I was delighted to see that even the NRC occasionally acknowledged that their test was unreliable and even considered the possibility of using treatment as a test. What is incomprehensible is that if you call the NRC to report that you have a Lyme patient who is seronegative, they will tell you this cannot be true because their test is perfect. Go figure!

Why is this empiric treatment, used as a diagnostic tool, not recommended for clinical presentations of Lyme disease other than for acute neurologic forms? 'Experts' probably have fewer scruples when it comes to less dramatic forms of the disease for which the risk of death or major disability is lower or takes longer to appear. Yet, in some recognised infectious diseases, such as tuberculosis, this empiric treatment strategy is quite widespread and accepted; we know that a quarter to a third of diagnosed tuberculosis is never proven by the culture of the tuberculosis agent *Koch bacillus*. The response to treatment is regarded as diagnostic.

In fact, again, very fortunately for patients, some clinicians do not hesitate to diagnose Lyme disease in seronegative patients with a very suggestive clinical picture, provided other possible diagnoses have been ruled out. In a major clinical trial on Lyme disease patients conducted in the United States by Klempner and colleagues, the results of which were published in 2001 in the prestigious *New England Journal of Medicine,* 40% of the patients included were seronegative.[122] Those patients had a history of erythema migrans, neurological or cardiac symptoms, arthritis and/or 'radiculoneuropathy' (nerve root damage). Unfortunately, the vast majority of clinicians, often unaware of the diagnostic difficulties associated with Lyme disease, prefer to make a commonly accepted but poorly substantiated diagnosis, often even without any evidence, such as: 'viral', 'autoimmune', 'degenerative', 'inflammatory', 'idiopathic' or (worst of all) 'psychosomatic'.

The importance of directly isolating responsible microbes

Blood serum testing is an indirect method – that is, it does not directly identify the microbe involved, but seeks to see if the patient has made antibodies against a particular microbe. An indirect method often requiring statistical trade-offs for its calibration, it is not always a 100%-reliable diagnostic method in infectious diseases. This is well known for some infections but too many doctors still give it a quasi-religious value.

To cite an example in the register of infections due to intracellular bacteria, I saw, a few years ago, a woman of Algerian origin who had gone to see her family in their village during the summer holidays. There, she had been in contact with dogs. When she returned to France in September, she showed all the characteristic signs of Mediterranean spotted fever, with high temperatures, violent headaches, a typical spotted rash and severe heart and lung damage. This disease, caused by *Rickettsia* bacteria, is transmitted by tick bites. She even had, in the fold of her groin, the 'black spot' characteristic of this disease. This black-crusted lesion corresponds to the bite site. Her antibody test for *Rickettsia conorii* remained hopelessly negative, even in Didier Raoult's laboratory in Marseille which has the reputation of having the best blood antibody test for *Rickettsia*. Likewise, amoebic abscess of the liver, and cysticercosis (a serious cerebral complication due to the *Taenia tapeworm* of the pig) are often associated with a negative antibody test. These are just a few examples. Antibody testing is imperfect.

Diagnostic issue 2: There are many different species of *Borrelia*

The bacterium originally described as the sole cause of Lyme disease is now called *Borrelia burgdorferi sensu stricto* (meaning 'strictly defined'). The prevalence of ticks infected with this bacterium varies greatly from one region to another. The prevalence is usually low, but there are high-risk areas. In Eastern Europe, 'hot spots' have been reported in which 40% of ticks have been found to be infected. In Alsace, 30% of ticks have been found to be infected in certain places. In the forest of Sénart, near Paris, 20% of ticks are infected. However, there are in fact a wide variety of species of *Borrelia* that can be implicated as the cause of Lyme disease. A broader group of bacteria have thus been described as the complex *Borrelia burgdorferi sensu lato* (meaning 'broadly defined'), which includes *Borrelia burgdorferi sensu stricto, Borrelia afzelii* and *Borrelia garinii.* In reality, the variety is even greater because these species themselves present a genetic diversity.

Since this classification was made, other species of *Borrelia* have regularly been isolated in different parts of the world. Some of these species have been isolated from patients with signs and symptoms identical or similar to those of Lyme disease: *Borrelia bavariensis, Borrelia bisettii, Borrelia valaisiana, Borrelia americana, Borrelia andersonii, Borrelia lonestari* and, more recently, *Borrelia kurtenbachii. Borrelia spielmanii* has been isolated in early skin lesions. The pathogenic role of *Borrelia lusitaniae,* isolated in a case of inflammation of the arteries, called vasculitis, remains to be substantiated. Recently, experts have included an even larger number of *Borrelia* species in the complex *Borrelia burgdorferi sensu lato,* even proposing to create a new genus, *Borreliella.*

Despite this diversity of strains, most commercially available tests still rely, as we have seen, on the original *Borrelia burgdorferi* strain B31 isolated in 1982 from a tick in the north east of the

United States (Shelter Island). A few years ago, at a congress, I asked Professor Benoît Jaulhac, the Director of the National Reference Centre (NRC) for Borreliosis, why he did not seek to develop tests to diagnose these numerous borrelioses. I told him about the numerous published case reports of diseases during which various *Borrelia species* had been isolated and deplored the fact that, for lack of study, we had no idea of their frequency in human pathology. He answered that this research would not really be useful since it was 'well-known' that these bacteria were poorly pathogenic in humans!

A new one: Borrelia miyamotoi

Previously unknown *Borreliae* continue to be discovered regularly. Thus, *Borrelia miyamotoi,* which has a Japanese name because it was recently discovered in Japan, is part of the group of *Borreliae* responsible for relapsing fevers: in addition to these fevers, it has the peculiarity of being able to cause syndromes identical to Lyme disease. In cases of relapsing fever, there is a high fever of 39° or 40°C, resembling a malaria attack, which disappears spontaneously and then returns iteratively for a variable period, sometimes prolonged over several years. Recently, this *Borrelia miyamotoi* has been found to be present throughout the Eurasian continent and in North America. Diseases of *Borrelia miyamotoi* (relapsing fever or Lyme) have been reported in Japan, Siberia, the Netherlands and the United States. This 'new' *Borrelia* has also been found in ticks in Alsace, the Ardennes and near Paris in the forest of Sénart. Despite this worldwide published knowledge, the NRC for Borreliosis in Strasbourg has been slow to develop a diagnostic tool for the detection of this organism.

In 2020, I published with Professor Michel Franck, a former teacher and researcher at the Lyon Veterinary School, and with other colleagues, the world's largest series of cases of *Borrelia miyamotoi* infection in French patients suffering from syndromes similar to chronic Lyme disease. Some of these patients had recurrent episodes of fever, as observed in relapsing fevers.[4] A Russian team previously reported, from patients living in Siberia, a large series of acute *Borrelia miyamotoi* infection occurring shortly after a tick-bite.[119]

The Sénart forest, in the Paris region, is a high-risk area. Indeed, this forest was contaminated by a charming squirrel, with beautiful stripes on its back, called the 'Korean squirrel'. This squirrel, which also bears the pretty name of 'bouroundouk', actually comes from Siberia and is therefore also called the 'Siberian tamia'.

This small beast with a charming appearance, resembling the squirrels of Walt Disney movies, was bought as a pet by private individuals. However, it is a wild creature that is unhappy in captivity and can become aggressive with children who try to play with it. Disconcerted by this very natural behaviour, the originally happy owners, who then became unhappy, released these animals into the Sénart forest. The Korean squirrels liked their new habitat and proliferated. The problem is that they harbour many more ticks than do their French counterparts and, moreover, their ticks have rates of infestation by *Borrelia* above the national average and close to those observed in Alsace.

The most recent one: Borrelia mayonii

In February 2016, a team from the north eastern United States described a new species implicated in Lyme disease cases. They suggested the name *Borrelia mayonii*. In the *Borrelia* genus, this *is* certainly not the last. Indeed, new bacterial species and variants of these species are regularly identified on all continents. For these multiple varieties, there is unfortunately no diagnostic test.

Diagnostic issue 3: Some so-called 'Lyme' cases may be caused by microbes other than *Borrelia*

Many microbes, sometimes transmitted by ticks and sometimes not, including bacteria and parasites and possibly some viruses, may be involved in conditions resembling Lyme, but we have no diagnostic tools to detect them currently. Among patients with early Lyme disease in the United States, 2–12% have been found also to have been infected with another bacterium – *Anaplasma* – responsible for the condition 'human granulocytic anaplasmosis'. Another 2–40% have been found to have babesiosis, a parasitic disease caused by a micro-organism of the piroplasmosis group, which is widespread in wild and domestic animals. Multiple infections may be the rule, not the exception.

Babesiosis, a major partner for Borreliae

Babesiae are parasites close to *Plasmodia*, the infective agents of malaria. They cause a malaria-like disease in animals that attacks red blood cells and is known as piroplasmosis. ('Piro' comes from the fact that these parasites are pear-shaped, not to be confused with 'pyro' meaning fever). This disease is called babesiosis in humans. In the countryside, all animals – dogs, cats, cows, horses, etc – that live outside in nature may develop piroplasmosis. These animals become tired, can have 'red urine' disease, lose weight and become feverish, anaemic and rheumatic. Farmers and vets are very familiar with this disease. Many such animals are treated regularly by vets. This disease is transmitted by ticks.

The same ticks bite humans and therefore inoculate them with *Babesiae* also. Officially, humans are resistant and do not develop this disease except in cases of profound immunosuppression or when they no longer have a functioning spleen (because it has been removed or because a disease has disrupted its functioning). In animals, we commonly see *Babesiae (Babesia divergens* and *Babesia microti*) in red blood cells by examining a drop of blood under the microscope. In humans, it is seen only in the rare situations mentioned above. Indeed, any infected red blood cells in healthy humans are filtered by the spleen and are not seen in the circulating blood. Not seeing *Babesiae* does not mean that they are not present; they can be hidden in certain tissues. Today, indirect diagnostic tests, such as antibody tests, are often unreliable. Many patients with chronic Lyme disease react strongly to some antiparasitic drugs and it is possible that *Babesiae* or other parasites have something to do with this.

Ticks also transmit other microbes...

Ticks can also transmit different *Bartonella* species, as well as other bacteria: *Ehrlichia chaffeensis* (in the United States), *Anaplasma phagocytophilum* (in mainland Europe), various *Rickettsia* species and *Francisella tularensis* (the agent causing tularaemia).

In Brazil, a disease close to Lyme, following an *Amblyomma* tick bite, has been described. Mobile spirochetes (spiral-shaped bacteria) have been seen in the blood of patients examined with dark field microscopy (looking into the microscope, mobile bacteria are visible on a dark background). However, contrary to some other spirochetes, including some species of *Borrelia,* microbiologists have not succeeded in isolating them by culture, despite using a variety of techniques.

A new pathogenic bacterium linked to tick bites, *Neoehrlichia mikurensis,* has been discovered in rats and ticks in Japan and then in humans in Sweden and Switzerland.[82] A Swedish publication showed that this 'new' bacterium had been found in a series of immunocompromised patients (suffering from lymphomas or autoimmune diseases) with signs and symptoms labelled as 'non-infectious', including serious cardiovascular events.[102] This bacterium is now suspected of being the cause of malignant lymphomas.

An antibiotic, doxycycline, is active against this bacterium. Some patients have been treated in several countries, with at least short-term efficacy.[180] In 2020, no large controlled study has been launched to demonstrate long-term efficacy of treatments. It is well known that this infection does not exist in France, Great Britain or Ireland… but then no medical microbiologist is looking for it! The only small concern is that once again the veterinary microbiologists are two lengths ahead of the medics: we now find this bacterium, just like *Borrelia miyamotoi,* is in ticks collected in French forests. But it is also well known that the French ticks do not bite French people! Why develop diagnostic tests for humans? This emerging bacterium has been found in ticks in Austria, Belgium, Czechia, Denmark, Estonia, France, Germany, Hungary, Italy, Moldova, Norway, Poland, Romania, Russia (Baltic regions), Serbia, Slovakia, Spain, Sweden, Switzerland and the Netherlands, but it has not been looked for yet in Great Britain or Ireland.[180]

These recent historical, geographical and microbial findings should prompt the medical community to understand that cases of chronic post-tick-bite syndromes are probably due to multiple pathogens and that these 'crypto-infections' require not only a new approach and but also a real paradigm shift in diagnosis and treatment.

Insights from veterinary medicine

One day, a sick woman of about 60 years of age, who was a sculptor living in Provence, came to see me for a chronic syndrome which included chronic fatigue, diffuse pains and especially pains in her upper abdomen that sounded excruciating when she described them. Her description resembled the atrocious pains of patients with severe pancreatic disease. She explained to me that she had been sick since childhood. At that time, she had lived in Gap in the Alps and everything started suddenly after an attack of acute pancreatitis 'came out of the blue'. Her pancreatitis had healed but the pains had never left her all her life.

All food intake was an ordeal for her because it caused flare ups and she had difficulty withstanding oral medication. Over the decades it had been going on she had consulted countless doctors, all of whom had told her the pain was in her head. To please some of these doctors, she had swallowed, when she could swallow, impressive amounts of analgesics and neuroleptics. Nothing had improved her symptoms. She spent part of each day in an analgesic position – that is, sitting with her torso bent forward on her thighs, a position in which she felt less pain. I was a little confused by her story which partly evoked chronic Lyme, but which was far from being typical. At that time, I was in contact with a Spanish veterinary microbiologist from Madrid who was looking for bacteria and parasites by polymerase chain reaction (PCR), the technique mentioned earlier. Faced with the negligence of medical microbiology laboratories, this veterinary biologist did offer his services from time to time to humans to carry out diagnostic tests. We had to whisper this, as it was frowned upon by some authorities – it seems we humans are not animals.

Despite this, the World Health Organization (WHO) supports the concept of 'One health' for people and animals on our planet, as we must learn to live together because we share the same environment, including the microbial environment. Vets have always been far ahead in the field of 'crypto-infections', but this fact is not going down well with some.

This patient sent a tube of blood to the veterinary biologist, without saying anyting about her symptoms. She just mentioned that the sample was 'from Professor Perronne'. I subsequently received a letter from this Spanish laboratory informing me that they had found in her blood by PCR *Borrelia burgdorferi* and an unidentified species of *Brucella*. *Brucellae* are known to be the cause of brucellosis, an animal disease (found in sheep, goats, cattle, etc) transmissible to humans, mainly through the consumption of unpasteurised milk or cheese. This disease is practically never seen in France now because all the contaminated livestock were slaughtered a long time ago. This infection is heavily monitored by vets among livestock but we know that the disease is currently coming back a little in certain regions, from wild animals.

Brucellosis was still rampant in the Alps when this woman was a child. I wrote to her, informing her of the test results. I got her to have an antibody blood serum test for brucellosis, which was done using the official techniques, but, as with her Lyme test, the result was negative. (At the time I received my medical training, seronegative brucellosis was not spoken of although we still often saw people with symptoms of brucellosis in our hospitals. I later learned that seronegative brucellosis not only exists but is also not uncommon. We must have missed a lot of cases in the past.)

I informed this patient that she had, provided there was no error in the Spanish lab (which was always possible), not only chronic Lyme disease, but also probable chronic brucellosis.

When I spoke to her about brucellosis, her face lit up and she asked me if it was the same thing as 'Maltese fever'. I confirmed this other name for the disease and she told me: 'When I was little and I was hospitalised for my pancreatitis, my father was hospitalised at the same time for Maltese fever that was cured and from which he recovered'. I was very impressed to see that a veterinary laboratory in Spain, without any clinical information and even less information about her family history, had hit the nail on the head.

I offered this woman a three-month course of antibiotic therapy, as recommended for brucellosis, with antibiotics also active against *Borrelia.* She had trouble swallowing the medicines, but her clinical condition improved rapidly, and her pain decreased. When she came to see me again at my clinic with her husband, she placed a beautiful sculpture on my desk representing a woman bent forward in an analgesic position. I was very moved that she had made this work for me. She said to me: 'I made this sculpture for you and I offer it to you because it symbolises the pancreatic pain I have had for almost 50 years. In my whole life you are the first doctor I have met who believed I was in pain.'

More reliable tools are needed to better identify causes of disease

Faced with the institutional denial of diseases caused by crypto-infections, leading an incalculable number of patients into the throes of hell, new techniques are essential to determine precisely what these patients are suffering from. The current situation, where imprecise testing methods are wrongly relied upon, not only leads to the misdiagnosis of many individual patients, but also has epidemiological consequences, via a general underestimation of the incidence of these diseases in all countries worldwide.

Tests using Scottish Borreliae *are more reliable than those made with the American reference* Borrelia

During a stay in London, where I attended a conference on chronic Lyme disease, I met English doctors who were following cases of this condition. If you look at official statistics, Lyme disease is even rarer in Britain than on the Continent. Several of these doctors were in trouble with the NHS because they were prescribing treatments for seronegative patients – 'fake patients' according to this organisation. Yet these British patients usually had very suggestive clinical signs of the disease, including a tick bite, an erythema migrans, and then various signs and symptoms affecting several body systems. A Scottish researcher, Mavin, struck by the very high proportion of negative antibody tests in British patients, wondered if this finding did not come from the fact that, worldwide, tests were being carried out with the historical American strain B31.

To investigate this, he took some negative serum samples from his freezer and repeated exactly the same antibody technique but replaced the American imposed strain B31 with Scottish *Borreliae*. Bingo, some serum samples turned out actually to be positive (Mavin et al, 2007, 2009). Patients were allowed back into the 'real patients' box again. It is likely that the British Isles, due to their geographical isolation, have different variants of *Borreliae* from the Continent. Perhaps this could explain why Lyme is never diagnosed in Corsica, another island where many undiagnosed symptomatic patients actually exist.

Even ticks are better off than humans when it comes to diagnostic tests

Veterinarians and entomologists (creepy-crawly specialists) are luckier than doctors because they can get funding to study tick microbes while infectious disease specialists are not entitled to any research funding for human patients (except for the frozen mummy of Ötzi, a late Neolithic man, that we will discuss later – see page 82). In 2013 Muriel Vayssier-Taussat, director of research at INRA (the Institut National de la Recherche Agronomique) in Maisons-Alfort, and her team, were able, thanks to new-generation sequencing, to identify various bacteria from *Ixodes ricinus* ticks harvested in France (in Alsace and the Ardennes): *Anaplasma phagocytophilum, Bartonella henselae, Bartonella grahamii, Borrelia afzelii, Borrelia garinii, Borrelia burgdorferi, Borrelia miyamotoi, Neoehrlichia mikurensis, Ehrlichia canis, Rickettsia canadensis, Rickettsia felis and Rickettsia Helvetica.* The problem is that doctors do not have any routine tests for these bacteria in humans either.

Muriel and her team, with Philippe Raymond, a general practitioner who looks after many patients with chronic Lyme and to whom I had introduced her, were able to test the serum samples of patients suffering from chronic post-tick-bite clinical pictures (groups of symptoms). She found evidence for the presence of *Bartonellae* in patient blood samples. The species *Bartonella henselae,* well known in humans, has been isolated from a few patients, but most surprisingly this investigation also led to the isolation of species previously unknown in human disease: *Bartonella doshiae, Bartonella schoenbuchensis* and *Bartonella tribocorum.* Muriel Vayssier-Taussat's work could have been challenged by medical microbiologists because she is an agronomic researcher and not a doctor so she asked Didier Raoult's medical laboratory to 'retest' the serum samples. The 'agronomic' results were confirmed and published by Muriel and her team in 2016.[233] What a boost that was for recognition of 'crypto-infections'!

Recently, a vet and his wife, who were both sick and who had also both faced the denial and incompetence of the medical profession who were unable to treat them, decided – all their tests being negative – to pretend they were both dogs and to send their samples to a veterinary laboratory. Bingo! A microbiological diagnosis was immediately found. So, I advise patients who are abandoned by their doctor to disguise themselves as wolves or lambs and go to see a vet; it will be much more effective.

In an article published in 2016, Muriel Vayssier-Taussat and Sara Moutailler and their team, presented a beautiful study on the microbial composition of French ticks collected from the Ardennes: a real pathogen zoo![233] Half of the ticks had been found to harbour at least one microbe that was pathogenic to humans, and half of those that were infected harboured several microbes. They found – hang on tight – the following:

- bacteria: *Borrelia garinii, Borrelia afzelii, Borrelia valaisiana, Borrelia burgdorferi sensu stricto, Borrelia miyamotoi,*

Borrelia spielmanii, Bartonella henselae, Rickettsia sp. of the spotted fevers group, mainly *Rickettsia helvetica, Anaplasma phagocytophilum* and *Neoehrlichia mikurensis;*
- parasites: *Babesia divergens.*

In addition, the following symbiotes, true cell 'parasites', were isolated: *Midichloria mitochondrii* and DNA sequences of *Wolbachia sp., Spiroplasma sp.* and *Acinetobacter sp.*

Bacteria belonging to the *Rickettsiae* type are the bacteria that most closely resemble our mitochondria – the micro-structures in our cells that produce energy. *Midichloria mitochondrii,* mentioned above, identified only recently, is a symbiotic bacterium capable of living in mitochondria but also of destroying them. Its possible role in animal or human pathology is still uncertain. The clinical signs of patients suffering from mitochondrial diseases resemble those of chronic Lyme. We are beginning to discover a new world.

Chapter 3

The certainties of a handful of experts in a world of uncertainties

The more you dig into the Lyme disease field, the more you realise that everything is opaque. Let us begin our descent into hell in the fog. Watch your step!

The gap between scientific publications and official recommendations

The most influential 'pseudo-experts' in the field we are dealing with appear to be able to neither read nor hear, but they talk, and the sick pay the price. It is worth noting that for two infectious diseases whose emergence was reported almost at the same time, Lyme disease at the end of the 1970s and the HIV-AIDS at the beginning of the 1980s, everything moves on in the field of HIV every day whereas everything is frozen without any evolution in the Lyme field. A major difference in the approach to the two diseases is that the funding for HIV infection research and management, from the very beginning of the AIDS pandemic, has been huge worldwide.

At the beginning of the AIDS epidemic, when the first Elisa test procedures were developed, the diagnosis of HIV infection was missed for a large proportion of patients because the sensitivity of the test was insufficient. When the Western blot antibody test became available, it was a great relief to see that it had now become possible to diagnose almost all HIV-infected patients. A few years later, I remember that one serotype of the HIV virus, serotype O, present in some parts of Africa, escaped commercialised testing. Immediately, the scientific community reacted to improve the tests. Currently, HIV serum antibody tests are hyper-reliable.

By contrast, if we take a look at the evolution of Lyme disease practices, attitudes have been different. An Elisa antibody test was again developed. Its lack of sensitivity has been widely published on, as I have said already. Many patients from whom the *Borrelia burgdorferi* bacterium was isolated in culture and whose serum antibody test nevertheless remained completely negative have been reported in scientific publications, including the most reputable international medical journals. This never appeared to concern the 'experts' who produced the recommendations on the disease. More seriously, when a more sensitive Western blot test was developed, its use as a first-line test was banned. As I have said above, it can be used only if the Elisa test proves positive. Curiously it is the only example of an infectious disease for which there is such a ban!

If we now look at the therapeutic side, we see that research on HIV treatment moved forward at an extraordinary pace, enabling us to arrive at highly effective triple-therapy regimens as early as the 1990s. In the field of Lyme, on the other hand, a handful of experts still refuse to read the many publications that show that *Borreliae* can survive several months of antibiotics; they continue to insist more than 30 years later that three weeks of antibiotic treatment can cure everyone. Meanwhile, hundreds of thousands of Lyme patients in North America and Europe have continued to deteriorate after having this 'official' treatment, to the point that many are in wheelchairs. The official IDSA recommendations published in 2006 completely ignore the most significant research and continue to convey the same simplistic discourse with some of the language we have already pointed out. It can be summed up in three cardinal assertions:

> Lyme is a rare disease.
>
> If one is infected, one will be cured with two to three weeks of penicillin.
>
> Chronic Lyme does not exist and all the patients who still have the impudence to complain of symptoms after treatment are mad and must be sent for psychiatric care.

What has happened in my home country, France, is instructive. In 2006, we copied the American recommendations, without questioning them; then in 2016 those recommendations were rejected by the National Guidelines Clearing House in the United States.

At the same time, the French Infectious Disease Society (la Société de Pathologie Infectieuse de Langue Française (SPILF)), decided to organise the Consensus Conference of 2006 that I mentioned earlier, at which the manipulation of the calibration of antibody tests I described in Chapter 2 was revealed during a tragi-comic episode. Professor Daniel Christmann of the University Hospital of Strasbourg was asked to organise the conference, because of the high frequency of Lyme in Alsace. Daniel, being a friend of mine and knowing I was interested in the disease, kindly asked me to assist him. I had already participated in the organisation of several meetings of French experts and of consensus conferences, notably for osteoarticular infections, tuberculosis, ENT infections and lower respiratory infections. I had also been a member of the organising committee for the first European consensus conference on HIV and hepatitis B and C virus (HBV and HCV) co-infections.

However, it so happened that at that time I was treating a patient from Alsace, suffering from chronic Lyme disease, who had entered into a conflict with the medical team at Strasbourg University Hospital and with the French national health insurance scheme (Sécurité Sociale) which, once again, did not want to recognise his illness and took him for a faker. This patient expressed his anger in an Alsatian newspaper. While I had nothing to do with it, my colleagues from Strasbourg expressed their dissatisfaction to me. I was sorry about that unfortunate incident but as a result, I was no longer invited to participate in the organisation of the consensus conference as planned.

The problem of chronic Lyme was consequently avoided during the debates and in the written documentation of this conference. A few weeks before the conference, Daniel Christmann, with whom I had kept friendly relations, invited me to be the moderator of a session, which I accepted. The conference presented an idealised picture of Lyme disease, with no problems in diagnosis or treatment, and the reports from experts, published a few months later in 2007 in the journal *Médecine et Maladies Infectieuses,* took up, almost to the letter, the recommendations by the USA's IDSA (see page 292) that had just come out.

Lyme disease and the reign of censorship

As I am used to publishing in various medical fields, I discovered while I was interested in Lyme that any paper that did not go in the same direction as the 'recommendations' of the IDSA Lyme group had a hard time getting published: the door of all the major medical journals was closed. I had heard about such scientific censorship, worthy of the inquisition, before but I only fully grasped its magnitude when I wanted to start publishing on the subject of Lyme.

In accordance with the standard scientific publication system, the typescript submitted to the journal is sent by the editor-in-chief or one of the associate editors to two experts in the field for critical 'peer' review. Even if it is not always the case, this external peer evaluation is, usually, pretty fair.

When it comes to Lyme, all the reviewers recite the IDSA recommendations and systematically demolish your work, with arguments that have no scientific basis, to conclude that your contribution is worthless and should definitely not be published. Usually, the article rejection is quick. For one of my articles, for which the data were well backed up and difficult to contradict, it took five reviewers plus the editor to reject it, and I had to wait for more than five months to be advised to go elsewhere. Even in 2015 and 2016, I had regular testimonies from European and American researchers who were unable to publish their work, even though it was of excellent quality.

A few years ago, I myself was a reviewer for a renowned international journal for which I had to evaluate a remarkable and even impressive piece of work, in terms of quantity and quality of findings, demonstrating the persistence of *Borrelia burgdorferi.* I made some criticisms regarding the detail and presentation, but I recommended its publication. The journal went ahead and published this work demonstrating the persistence of *Borrelia* (which, as we have seen, does not exist according to IDSA) so I was stunned when the embarrassed editorial staff of the journal sent me a copy of a letter from a prominent member of the small IDSA clique, demanding the immediate withdrawal and cancellation of the article. The letter said this should be done because the persistence of *Borreliae* was not possible since their group had been proclaiming this was the case for decades. It seemed it was forbidden to publish scientific data if it was not in line with the official diktat even if the evidence was entirely to the contrary. This letter caused quite a stir among the editorial staff, but fortunately the journal did not give into the pressure and maintained the publication which is now a reference.

A world of 'certainties' is beginning to show some cracks

In 2011, under a headline including the word 'anti-science', Paul Auwaerter with a few of his colleagues wrote an astonishing and terrifying article equating patients with chronic Lyme disease with lunatics, and doctors who treated them with charlatans in the journal *Lancet Infectious Diseases*,[31] making unfounded connections with the worst examples of bad medical practice, including anti-vaccine movements. As I was very shocked by this text, which included violent accusations that were not based on any solid scientific data, I sent a letter of response to the journal which it was decent enough to publish in 2012.[16]

I was saddened when, shortly afterwards, *Lancet Infectious Diseases* published a 'response to the responses' in which Professor Didier Raoult, a microbiologist in the Faculty of Medicine, Aix-Marseille University, Marseille, affirmed that chronic Lyme was an invention created by patients suffering from unexplained disorders and that the internet served as a sounding board for these misguided discussions.[187] He claimed, in passing, that the Western blot diagnostic test had no value, compared with the Elisa test, for Lyme disease (which, as we have seen, has been contradicted by many publications as well as by the latest CDC diagnostic criteria in the United States). All this, he added, reminded him of the dubious practices of Charles Nicolle's students – namely Giroud and Jadin, father and daughter (not mentioned in the text, but this could be read between the lines by insiders) – who were the originators of the concept of 'chronic rickettsioses' that led to diagnostic tests for these conditions.

Cécile Jadin, who as I have said (see page 25) currently practises in South Africa, had followed in her father's footsteps. I do not know if Willy Burgdorfer, who was still alive at the time, followed these exchanges in *Lancet Infectious Diseases*, but if he did, he must have been deeply sorry to see the stand taken by this well known researcher who succeeded him as head of the World Health Organization Reference Centre for Rickettsiosis.

I don't bear Didier Raoult any ill will – indeed, I think highly of him – but I would very much like him to help patients and the medical community by improving research in this field. Indeed, even if he is not convinced that *Borrelia burgdorferi* and/or the *Rickettsiae* are responsible for chronic conditions, there are all the other microbes responsible for 'crypto-infections' to look for. Even for the *Rickettsiae*, chronic forms of infection have been described: for example, Brill–Zinsser disease, a persistent and relapsing form of epidemic typhus, caused by *Rickettsia prowazekii*. It is meanwhile noteworthy that Paul Auwaerter, who described the chronic form of Lyme disease as 'anti-science' in 2011, was to publish articles praising the effectiveness of many compounds, either chemical or herbal, against the 'persistent forms of *Borrelia*' three years later, in 2014,[84] and then again in 2015[85] and also in 2016.[89]

These later articles are excellent; I could not believe my eyes when I read them and I checked very carefully that the author was not a different researcher with the same name. Of course, given his seniority, he was not the first author and his name was simply added to the work done by many other researchers, including Jie Feng and Ying Zhang. Nevertheless, I was astonished to see that this man was able to change his mind so quickly and to affirm unreservedly the opposite of what he had categorically asserted before. Indeed, it is this same Dr Auwaerter who has since published two editorials attacking the very idea of chronic Lyme.[31, 152] I don't mind if people change their minds once, but please, not every year!

In order to understand this scientific imbroglio, this misinformation and *omerta*, we have to go back in time, which we will do in the next chapter.

Chapter 4

The history of ticks and spiral-shaped bacteria

Our human cells, like all animal cells, are derived from bacteria – primitive unicellular beings. Bacteria and other microbes have evolved over billions of years; they have gradually adapted to the environment, combining or exchanging genetic material to create increasingly complex structures, including animal cells. Some 'useful' bacteria have even been permanently incorporated by animal and therefore human cells. This is how mitochondria – energy-producing sub-components of our cells – allow us to survive in oxygen and even to use it. From the remarkable work by Sagan and Margulis, *Microcosmos* (1986), we learn that mobile spiral-shaped bacteria in the form of small springs, called 'spirochetes', have played, and continue to play, a major part in the evolution of animal and human species. Spirochetes provided the basic microtubular structure of our cells. Knowing this, it is less surprising that other spirochetes can hide easily within our cells and that their presence can disrupt their functioning all the more easily as they have so many points in common with them.

Spiral-shaped bacteria

Lyme disease is due, as I described earlier, to the bacterium *Borrelia burgdorferi* that is shaped like a small spiral or spring, as are other species of *Borreliae*. These spiral-shaped bacteria belong in particular to the order of spirochetales, class of spirochetes. Humans and other animals have always lived together with many microbes and in particular these spirochetes. While the ancestors of spirochetes helped to shape our cells, today's spirochetes are mobile bacteria that can move through the body's biological fluids and cause many ailments. Thus, spirochetes are associated with many 'crypto-infections'. 'Borrelioses' are infectious diseases caused by the *Borreliae* family of spirochetes and most often transmitted, as we have seen, by vectors, the most common being lice and ticks depending on the species of *Borrelia*. Most species of bacteria have an animal reservoir (birds, rodents or other mammals).

There are many spiral-shaped bacteria

Spiral-shaped bacteria are not limited to spirochetes, and spirochetes are not limited to the *Borreliae*. The spirochete class includes other bacterial types such as *Treponema* and *Leptospira*. The most famous treponemus is *Treponema pallidum*, or 'pale treponema', the infective agent of syphilis, a sexually transmitted disease that ravaged the world for centuries. It was called 'pale' because it was not coloured by usual stains used for looking at cells under a microscope.

Leptospirosis is a disease that is caught by contact with the urine of contaminated rodents, particularly through small skin wounds, on the shores of lakes or rivers in summer. Leptospirosis is most often benign, but severe and even fatal forms of it are possible in the absence of antibiotic treatment.

Another spiral bacterium that has become famous is *Helicobacter pylori* of the order of Campylobacterales, family Helicobacteraceae. *Helicobacter pylori* has recently been recognised as the agent of gastric and duodenal peptic ulcer disease, which for over a century had been considered a psychosomatic condition. Interestingly, as early as 1875, German researchers, whose observations were to be confirmed in 1900 by French researchers, had noticed the presence of spiral-shaped bacteria in the stomach, and especially in ulcers, but it was believed that these bacteria passed through these regions because of the inflammation present in the ulcer and could in no way be responsible and even less survive in the very acidic environment of the stomach. The discovery of the relationship between ulcer and bacteria was linked to a 'laboratory error', as is often the case (as in the discovery of penicillin).

In Australia, Barry Marshall, a young gastroenterologist in training in Robin Warren's department, was in charge of culturing gastric biopsies. He failed 34 times to grow bacteria because he was, as is usual, monitoring the result of his cultures at 48 hours. At the 35th try, he forgot his culture boxes during the long Easter weekend. Result: five days later, the bacteria that would later be named *Helicobacter pylori* had grown.

This significant discovery did not convince the medical community in Australia or elsewhere; Marshall's work was systematically denigrated, and he and Warren were prevented from publishing their results for a long time. In the face of the jibes of official medicine, Marshall courageously had to swallow a test-tube of bacteria in front of witnesses, develop a stomach ulcer in less than a week and then heal his ulcer with antibiotics so that he could be believed. As just reward, he and his colleague received the Nobel Prize for Physiology or Medicine in 2005. It is interesting to see that now *Helicobacter pylori* specialists can analyse genetic variants of the bacterium to study human migrations in history. A recent study published by Tan in 2015 also showed a link between *Helicobacter pylori* infection and the severity of Parkinson's disease.[227]

About 15 years ago, I sat on a commission of the French National Agency for Research on AIDS and Viral Hepatitis (ANRS), responsible for selecting research projects on infectious liver diseases. I was the only infectious disease specialist, surrounded by many hepato-gastroenterologists and some microbiologists. A French microbiologist had shown that other *Helicobacter* species (non-*pylori*) could be found in pieces of organs removed by surgeons from people suffering from various hepatobiliary pathologies (autoimmune primary biliary cirrhosis, alcoholic cirrhosis, sclerosing cholangitis, cancer, etc). He was asking for funding to continue his research. I found this theme fascinating but unfortunately, I was the only one in the room to think so. For hepato-gastroenterologists, looking for bacteria as the origin of diseases was out of the question. There were a lot of other more serious things to fund in their view!

I thought, saddened, that perhaps they had not yet properly digested the blow to their assumptions caused by the discovery of *Helicobacter pylori* as the cause of stomach ulcers. For the specialty, the progressive disappearance of this disease has meant a loss in earnings. The follow-up of ulcers meant a lifelong income with regular endoscopies to check on developments. The presence of *Helicobacter* non- *pylori* in the stomach has, however, been described.[64] Meanwhile, the processes that cause the liver to become fibrous and hard (fibrosis then cirrhosis) have not been fully elucidated. The liver is a very large organ that filters blood downstream from the digestive tract. It would not be surprising if 'tenants' of the liver – small microbes – increased the harmful effects of excessive alcohol or sugar consumption, or chronic hepatitis B or C viruses, recognised factors in the development of steatosis (fatty liver disease), cirrhosis and even liver cancer.

The *Borreliae*

The *Borreliae* began to be identified at the end of the nineteenth century though there was no way to culture them at the time. The name *Borrelia* was created in 1907 by the Swedish microbiologist Swellengrebel, who studied spirochetes and contributed to the recognition of *Treponema pallidum* as the cause of syphilis.

This was not so simple because some researchers still questioned the infectious origin of this famous venereal disease. For the church, it was convenient to continue to make it a divine punishment for the 'sins of the flesh'. Discovering spirochetes different from treponemas, he named them *'Borrelia'* in honour of his French colleague and friend, Amédée Borrel, a bacteriologist trained in Montpellier, who entered the Pasteur Institute in Paris in 1892 as a researcher, and was responsible for the microbiology course at the institute and co-founded the *Bulletin* of the Pasteur Institute.

After developing the first French gas mask during the First World War, Borrel settled in Strasbourg, which had returned to French rule in 1919. The first borrelioses he identified were relapsing fevers. One of these is of worldwide distribution and transmitted by human lice (*Pediculus humanus*), caused by *Borrelia recurrentis.* Like other louse-borne diseases – exanthematic typhus, for example – this relapsing fever is facilitated by poverty, migration and the coming together of populations in unhealthy conditions. This is why this disease emerges in war zones or in prison or refugee camps. It was recently shown by Didier Raoult's team that, during their retreat from Russia in 1812, Napoleon's louse-covered Great Army soldiers not only died of cold but were also killed in their thousands by diseases transmitted by lice: *Bartonella quintana,* the agent of trench fever, and *Rickettsia prowazekii,* the agent of exanthematic typhus.

Other relapsing fevers are limited to smaller geographical outbreaks and are transmitted by particular tick species. At least 15 species of *Borrelia* can cause relapsing tick fevers. In Africa, ticks of the *Ornithodoros* type are soft ticks responsible for massive infections in the population. These ticks are very often present in the cracks in the walls of houses where infected rodents hide. The best known *Borreliae* are *Borrelia crocidurae* in the Sahara and Sahel, *Borrelia duttonii* in East Africa and *Borrelia hispanica* in Spain and Northwest Africa. In Sahel, it is well established in published studies that a high proportion of cases of high-grade fever attributed to malaria are in fact borreliosis.[234, 149] Routinely, in the absence of tests, these borrelioses are never diagnosed. At the end of 2015, a French patient whose brother was in the Expeditionary Force in Mali was surprised that all the soldiers' high grade fevers were systematically labelled 'malaria' while many, according to his brother's observations of other soldiers, began their 'malaria' with an erythema migrans (the bull's-eye rash described earlier).

Yet these relapsing fevers and their link with ticks have been known for ages. Relapsing tick fever has been reported in Madagascar ('Malagasy fever') since Robert Drury wrote his memoirs *Madagascar: Robert Drury's Journal* in 1729. His book was very successful and was reprinted several times, although he was accused of embellishing his adventures and of copying some of them from the book *Histoire de la Grande Isle Madagascar (The History of the Big Madagascar Island)* by the French historian and explorer Etienne de Flacourt, published in 1661.

Drury, born in London in 1687, boarded the ship *Degrave* setting sail for India in 1701 as a young ship's boy. During the return journey, the ship sank off the coast of Madagascar. He made it to the shore but was taken prisoner by the local king and enslaved. After many adventures, in 1717, he managed to escape on an English ship sent by his father. He returned to London and went back to Madagascar as a pirate and slave merchant. Having witnessed wars between tribes, Drury reported that the Vazimba would have kept many *Ornithodoros* ticks in their homes to prevent their Sakalavian enemies from entering, which would have exposed them and inevitably made them contract the 'tick disease', while they themselves were probably immune from an early age (François Rodhain, Archives of the Pasteur Institute of Madagascar).

At the beginning of the twentieth century, 'Hispano-African relapsing fever' was described between the two world wars, and attributed to a spirochete called, at the time, *Spirochaeta hispanicum,* which was finally recognised as a *Borrelia.*

We are all made with microtubules from spirochetes in our cells

What part did spirochetes play in our evolution? To answer this question, Sagan and Margulis put forward some suggestive data. Spirochetes have always had the feature of being very mobile, thanks to their microtubular structures. This mobility has given them an advantage in microbial competition, allowing them to escape hostile environments or to gain areas rich in nutritive substances. Among the spirochetes, there were some very nasty ones capable of killing other cells to survive. Some friendlier spirochetes were able to help other microbes or motionless cells to move, by playing the role of a pusher. This contributed to the positive selection of some cells. Finally, other spirochetes, of the intermediate model, were able to enter cells, not to kill them, but to transform them from within and possibly take advantage of them while helping them to survive. Thus, a few million years ago, our cells, which were on the path to becoming animal and then human cells, were built from spirochete microtubules – small tubes allowing mobility but also many other functions in the cell, first in the bacterial cell then the animal and eventually human cell, like a construction game.

Our bodies are stuffed with spirochete microtubules. The cells of our respiratory system have undulating cilia that line our bronchi to bring impurities up to the larynx; the cilia undulate thanks to spirochete microtubules. Hormones are secreted in the body *via* spirochete microtubules – for example, insulin produced by the pancreas. Nerve cells are built on the basis of these microtubules, as are visual cells. The flagella of sperm that allow them to progress at high speed and throw themselves into women's fallopian tubes in a race to the egg, are made of these mobile microtubules. Even the microtubules arranged in beams that allow our chromosomes to split during the division of our cells – the process called 'mitosis' – are spirochete microtubules. Thinking about it makes the head spin but we can then understand better why, when small, apparently harmless, bacteria of the spirochete family enter our organs and cells, they are able to confuse the functioning of our own microtubules and thus disrupt the functioning of many things in the body.

Relapsing fever borreliosis is no longer routinely diagnosed in modern medicine

In the past, tropical disease physicians confirmed the diagnosis of borreliosis by microscopic blood smear tests, but this practice has fallen into disuse, and there is no longer any way to routinely diagnose these extremely common diseases in modern medicine. The only cases are diagnosed sporadically during research. This is all the more disturbing since, in developed countries, nearly half of all unexplained prolonged fevers have a clinical profile consistent with *Borrelia* relapsing fever.

Our tick friends – vectors of infections

Contrary to popular belief, ticks are not insects. Like insects, they are 'arthropods' (literally 'jointed limbs'), but belong to another family – the arachnids, which include spiders, dust mites (including chiggers), sarcoptes, and scorpions.

Among the many mechanisms of transmission of infectious diseases, the role of arthropod vectors is major. They can be arachnids but also insects, such as mosquitoes, lice or shield bugs, including the bug that transmits careotrypanosis (or Chagas' disease) in Latin America. These arthropods – mosquitoes, fleas, lice and ticks – have played, and continue to play, a major role in the history of animals and humans: they have been the cause of the greatest epidemics and pandemics (epidemics affecting several continents) that have decimated huge populations.

Ticks are usually regarded as less scary because we have seen them on various animals, including livestock and pets. A lot of people get bitten by ticks without realising it and without any apparent problems, at least at the time. Yet these seemingly harmless beings are formidable. There are hard ticks and soft ticks (mentioned above). Some are resistant like small armoured tanks; some can remain a year without eating or drinking. Through gene exchange, they certainly play a part in the evolution of species, but unfortunately, they also transmit many microbes that are responsible for infections. On the one hand, the diseases induced are acute, sometimes serious, but are often easily diagnosed. On the other hand, some diseases are latent and can become chronic; these 'silent infections' are poorly known.

Ticks are widespread in large numbers all over the planet. Even if they probably prefer to sink their rostrum (mouth parts) into a rat, doe or shrew, they are not choosy when a human passes nearby. They're like little vampires. The rostrum is a hollow, tapered structure that is used like a needle, containing some sub-structures that can cut the skin like small scissors and also some small anti-reverse hooks that allow the tick to hang on tightly, like a harpoon. Ticks operate very efficiently by giving a local anaesthetic and secreting a kind of glue that firmly secures the rostrum. Thanks to enzymes contained in their saliva, ticks will destroy tissues around the bite site, thus forming a small pocket of blood under the skin (or 'blood lake') by rupturing blood capillaries. The blood will mix with cellular debris and the tick's salivary secretions and the tick will not only feed, but also regurgitate into this pocket and thus transmit microbes.

There are different cycles depending on tick types and species. Hard ticks like their meals to last – they latch on for extended periods. For hard ticks of the *Ixodes* type, the duration of a meal is two to three days for larvae, about five days for nymphs and up to about 10 days for adult females. By gorging herself with blood, the female can increase her weight more than 600 times, and her size can exceed one centimetre in length. The adult male does not feed but mates with the female during her meal on the host. Then the male dies. The female drops off to lay her eggs, after which she dies in turn.

If the blood meal is shortened, the tick can resume it on a new host (in infectious disease terminology, victims are called 'hosts' because they house the germs free of charge). It is called a bite or sting because in fact the tick carries out both at the same time. Ticks love us very much. They are small, ultra-resistant, mobile syringes that feed on blood only three times in their lives, once at each stage of their life-cycle. The tick goes from larva to nymph then from nymph to adult. If you want to raise ticks at home, some are very cute, and they don't cost much to feed! The larva measures less than one millimetre and the nymph one to two millimetres. The larva can wait a year without eating. An adult tick can also fast for several months if an animal or human is not kind enough to pass by. Ticks can hydrate themselves by absorbing moisture from their surroundings. They like to wait for their prey in tall grasses or ferns and are particularly numerous in forests. They detect the heat and carbon dioxide emitted by their future victims. Some tick species are less passive and prefer to hunt and run to reach a victim. The painless sting can go unnoticed, especially if a tick bites in an area not easily accessible to the eye (the back, skin folds, navel, scalp, ear canal, buttock-line or genital lips).

Soft ticks are fast-food adepts and often fall off after a meal lasting a few minutes to a few hours. Some soft ticks can fast for five years. Being much smaller than adults, nymphs very often go unnoticed. Even if they are less full of *Borreliae* than adults, nymphs, being 10 to 50 times more numerous, are the major source of infection. Larvae are even smaller, but being 10 times less infected than nymphs, they transmit more rarely. It is understandable that the majority of people infected by ticks have no memory of a bite.

The many species of tick found around the world host an incalculable variety of microbes (bacteria, parasites and viruses). An international scientific publication was even entitled *The Tick Menagerie*. Fortunately, all these microbes do not cause diseases in humans, and tick infestation rates for a particular microbe are highly variable from one region to another. Ticks, having spent their time exchanging microbial genetic material with many animal species for millennia, including humans, probably play a part in the evolution of species.

Unfortunately, these 'exchanges' often result in the occurrence of diseases. If we look at history, many diseases that have decimated entire populations are transmitted by vectors such as mosquitoes (e.g. malaria), fleas (e.g. plague) or lice (e.g. typhus).

In many parts of the world, and particularly in Europe and North America, there has been a significant increase in the number of ticks in nature. Several factors could be involved in this increase. While deforestation may be a major problem in some parts of the world, the area covered by forests is expanding in Europe and North America. Hunters are less numerous and game is proliferating and comes into contact with dwellings. In other regions of the world, as habitat is destroyed and man encroaches, animals are forced into contact with people. Man-induced upheavals in nature have probably also reduced tick predator-animal populations. Global warming could play a part. Even though ticks remain more active in fine weather, tick bites with erythema migrans are being seen in the middle of winter in France. Moreover, ticks are travelling. For example, they are crossing Europe from east to west on trucks due to the importation of wild boars for hunting, or birds.

Others travel in hay bales. Ticks from cold, temperate or warm countries do not require the same temperatures for maximum activity as their native counterparts. Thus, a Scandinavian immigrant tick used to a cold climate could be having the time of its life in the middle of winter in France, Great Britain or Ireland.

Chapter 5

The history of Lyme disease

The disease in Europe

Amongst 'crypto-infections' Lyme disease stands as one of the earliest known and scientifically chronicled, yet its nature, indeed its very existence, has over the past half century met with a barrage of what can only be called unhelpful scepticism at best; and, at worst, an unaccountable degree of obstruction.

Although not yet so-named, the first descriptions of Lyme disease date back to the end of the nineteenth century in Europe. The connection between a tick bite and the initial, now classical, rash, which represents the primary stage of the disease, was in fact formally recorded over 100 years ago.

The later stages of the disease were described in the 1920s, when cases of meningeal and neurological disturbance, including paralysis, were reported following tick bites, first in France, then in Germany.

For decades, such tick-borne diseases were ill-managed and ill-understood, despite a considerable number of scientific voices suspecting, then asserting, that spirochetes – spiral-shaped bacteria, as described in the previous chapter – were the cause, and antibiotics an efficacious treatment.

It was not until the description of the American epidemic in the town of Old Lyme, Connecticut, in the 1970s, followed by the discovery of *Borrelia burgdorferi*, the bacterium responsible, that the disease found its name, and diagnostic tests were developed. Formal diagnosis, unfortunately, was limited to the patient's blood serum antibody status – and, as we have seen in earlier chapters, this testing regime was to constitute a major methodological obstacle to the identification and medical management of the illness.

In the late nineteenth and early twentieth centuries, medical practitioners (dermatologists, neurologists, rheumatologists, psychiatrists) observed, each within their respective fields and specialist associations, that patients could come to them with ill-health, in some cases severe, following a tick bite. Whilst the cause remained long unknown, attribution to spirochetes does appear in the scientific literature and, since the 1950s, the efficacy of antibiotics has been reported and documented. For decades, no connection was made between the different forms of the illness, due to the widely varying symptoms seen. This explains in part why, for so long, the disease did not have a formal, unifying name.

In 1910, Arvid Afzelius, a Swedish dermatologist, noted and reported the appearance of a red, ring-shaped lesion following a bite from a tick of the *Ixodidae* family. Lipschutz reported identical cases in Austria in 1913, for which he proposed the name 'erythema chronicum migrans' (ECM).

In 1922, two French physicians from Lyon, Charles Garin and Charles Bujadoux, described a form of meningo-radiculitis (an affliction of the nerve roots) that would bear their names. The first case was that of a child who had earlier presented with erythema migrans. Neurological manifestations were observed following a tick bite, with paralysis in some cases, which could be serious and occasionally fatal. Garin and Bujadoux were convinced, without managing to prove it, that such tick-related paralytic illness was caused by non-syphilitic spirochetes. Tantalisingly, in 1928 at Heidelberg University, Steiner identified non-syphilitic spirochetes in the brains of patients who had died of multiple sclerosis. And in 1930, Hellerström, in Sweden, confirmed the connection between some forms of meningitis and erythema migrans.

A connection was made retrospectively between the entity now known as Lyme disease and another cutaneous syndrome described in Breslau, Germany, in 1883, by Dr Alfred Buchwald. This condition consisted of chronic skin problems characterised by premature ageing of the skin, which took on a parchment-like appearance, most conspicuously on the lower limbs. In 1894, Pick, followed by Herxheimer and Hartmann in 1902, described identical cases. Today this condition is known as acrodermatitis chronica atrophicans or Pick-Herxheimer syndrome.

The tragic fate of Karl Herxheimer, victim of the Nazis

Karl Herxheimer, a German national who we know of best today because of the so called 'Herx reaction' (see below), was one of the greatest dermatologists of his time. He had exceptional clinical experience in all aspects of syphilitic infection and was also highly knowledgeable about this 'new disease', yet to be named 'Lyme disease'. Karl Herxheimer died on 6th December 1942 at Theresienstadt concentration camp in the Sudetenland, a region now part of Czechia.

Before he was killed, it seems that the breadth of his medical and scientific knowledge had come to the attention of Nazi scientists in charge of researching tick-transmitted diseases, most notably the celebrated veterinary scientist, Erich Traub. The latter had undertaken a research internship before the war at the Rockefeller Institute for Medical Research in Princeton, New Jersey, under the supervision of Richard Shope. Returning to Germany during the Second World War, Traub worked on the development of microbiological weapons on the island of Riems in the Baltic Sea, near Greifswald, in the German region of Mecklenburg-West Pomerania. This research centre had been created in 1910 by Friedrich Löffler, before being diverted from its initial purpose by the Third Reich. Traub was Vice-President of the Friedrich Löffler Institute. Human diseases transmitted by arthropods (insects and arachnids) were also extensively studied on human 'guinea pigs' at the Institut für Entomologie (Entomology Institute) set up at Dachau concentration camp in Bavaria.

Years before his tragic death at the age of 81, Karl Herxheimer, with his Austrian colleague Adolf Jarisch, had recorded and described the occasionally violent exacerbation of symptoms during treatment of syphilis with mercury salts. The designation Jarisch-Herxheimer reaction (or 'Herx' to the initiated) was given to this reaction, frequently observed at the onset of treatment – a collision, as it were, between treatment and disease, often also called a 'die off' reaction. Whilst this was first described in the context of mercury treatment for syphilis, it was later reported following the administration of antibiotic agents in syphilitic patients. Mercury treated the infection but, being a toxic, heavy metal, its administration led to complications of a highly noxious nature. At the time, it was quipped that 'syphilitics fall from the arms of Venus into those of Mercury', in time predicating a switch from mercury treatment of syphilitic patients to antibiotics. Later, analogous reactions were described during the treatment of Lyme disease.

Further European research into the disease

In 1943, in Sweden, Bo Bäfverstedt described 'lymphadenosis benigna cutis'. Earlier, and following Garin and Bujadoux, in 1941, Bannwarth had also reported a form of meningitis following a tick bite. From then onwards, the disease fell under various names: Garin-Bujadoux syndrome, Bannwarth syndrome or Garin-Bujadoux-Bannwarth syndrome. Another skin lesion, characteristic of the disease but less frequent, was benign cutaneous lymphocytoma, described in 1911 by Burckhardt. Bäfverstedt gave it its name in 1943. Nowadays it is known as 'borrelial lymphocytoma' – an inflammatory and tender lesion often resembling a small red ball on a patient's earlobe or, less frequently, the nipple or scrotum. We now know, thanks to Eva Sapi's research published in 2016, that such lymphocytomas contain sheets ('biofilms') of *Borrelia.*

In 1948, in Germany, Carl Lenhoff identified spirochetes in biopsies but his results were attributed to artefacts – misleading results proceeding from faulty methods, it was said – and ignored. As often in science, when someone is the first to see something, others say it's impossible and their work is denigrated. In 1949, Hellerström also suggested spirochetes as the cause.

In 1949, Thyresson, in Sweden, in a study of 57 patients suffering from acrodermatitis chronica atrophicans, demonstrated the efficacy of penicillin. In 1951, Hollström, in Sweden, chronicled the potency of penicillin upon erythema chronicum migrans. Another study of 67 patients, published in 1953, further confirmed penicillin as effective in treating erythema chronicum migrans. In 1955, Binder and his colleagues in Germany, crucially reported that an infectious agent present in a case of erythema chronicum migrans, sensitive to penicillin, could be transmitted to humans through a tick of the *Ixodes ricinus* species. He was unable at the time to identify the organism. He was, however, able to confirm experimental transmission from human to human through material extracted from a zone of erythema chronicum migrans. This experimental transmission between human subjects was also demonstrated by Götz in 1954 from a case of acrodermatitis chronica atrophicans, and by Paschoud in 1958, from benign cutaneous lymphocytoma. At the time, experiments on humans evidently dispensed with ethics committees' approval!

Ötzi, first 'lymee' of the late Neolithic age

Proof that these bacteria have existed for a very long time is provided by the recent discovery, by ramblers in 1991, of what has come to be known as the 'mummy of Ötzi', in the Tyrolian Alps between Austria and Italy. This man, in all likelihood a hunter since he was carrying a dagger, a bow and arrows and a copper hatchet, died about 5300 years ago, at the end of the Neolithic era, during the copper age. For millennia his body remained frozen in a glacier but emerged following an exceptional ice-melt in the Alps. Unlike patients today, who have little access to reliable diagnostic tests, Ötzi saw substantial funds lavished upon research on his body.

Surprise, surprise – Ötzi's organs had played host to the scattered genome of a *Borrelia* subtype, 60% identical to that of *Borrelia burgdorferi*, the infective agent of Lyme disease – an inconvenient discovery in the face of the widespread opinion that this was a rare, emerging disease in Europe. Were one to believe the chorus of official voices in contemporary medicine, that intrepid hunter from the late Neolithic age happened upon one of the rare contaminated ticks lurking in Europe at the time. Strange and mysterious it is not, that the only frozen hunter identified from our Neolithic era should be carrying an infection related to Lyme disease.

Ötzi did not die of the disease. He was killed by an arrow, the head of which was embedded in his left shoulder, having pierced his subclavian artery. He sported tattoos in his lumbar region and over his knee and ankle joints, suggesting that he'd consulted a specialist of the time to treat his musculoskeletal problems – we know that therapeutic tattoos were common in those days. Ötzi was riddled with arteriosclerosis. He also believed in phytotherapy (herbal medicine): his knapsack contained medicinal mushrooms used at the time to treat certain parasites – a happy epoch, long before the Vichy government outlawed herbalism during the Nazi occupation of France, and more recently, before health authorities started suing phytotherapists for being charlatans.

Another strange historical twist lies in Ötzi's Corsican origins. The current official version would have us believe that Corsica is untouched by Lyme disease. My Corsican patients, infected by ticks in the Corsican scrub, do not subscribe to that view. Tick-borne diseases have existed throughout history. Noah's ark was probably teeming with infected ticks!

The disease in America

As outlined in Chapter 1, the disease acquired its current name from the town of Lyme in the American state of Connecticut, or more precisely, the small town of Old Lyme, situated close to the mouth of the Connecticut river. In native American Indian idiom, 'Connecticut' means 'long river'. This is the site of one of the oldest British settlements in the region, dating back to 1630–1640. Lyme is a small, quiet town set in greenery, full of beautiful houses, some in the British colonial style. A meticulously tended lawn adorns the front of the small First Congregational Church, founded in 1665. Since the seventeenth century, the population had lived happily in their tranquil paradise, perhaps a little too tranquilly, as in the 1970s misfortune fell upon the region.

The Connecticut river may be long and quiet, but life on its banks certainly didn't flow as tranquilly as one might have thought. Many people fell ill with great fatigue, complaining of a variety of health issues and aches and pains – particularly in their joints – as well as neurological and/or cardiac problems. In children, inflammation of the joints, or arthritis, was a particularly common symptom. At the time, doctors invariably diagnosed juvenile rheumatoid arthritis or Still's disease, an autoimmune condition known to rheumatologists but poorly understood in its fundamentals. 'Autoimmune' diseases are inflammatory disorders, the precise underpinnings of which are unknown, the theory being that the organism (human body in this case) turns against itself by activating its immune system against its own cells or tissues, instead of attacking germs or other intruders.

The saga of Lyme disease in America

The alarm was first sounded by a woman living in Lyme, Polly Murray, an artist and painter by profession. Polly had been ill since 1956, suffering from chronic fatigue, headaches, aches and pains in the joints and eczematous lesions. She attributed this to a pregnancy, and for a while, the symptoms seemed to ebb away. In 1965, her illness resumed more disruptively than ever, with, additionally, cognitive issues in the form of memory and concentration lapses. She consulted numerous doctors who assured her that her symptoms were psychosomatic. She was a hypochondriac, they said. One doctor even ventured: 'You know, Mrs Murray, some people nurture an unconscious wish to be ill'. She was referred to a psychiatrist. This is not untypical of many of our patients' experience. Nothing has changed in half a century.

Desperate and in failing health, Polly spent endless hours at the university library, trying in vain to identify the cause of her troubles. In the early 70s, her older son fell ill; in time, her younger boy did too. They had very similar symptoms and both had had red circular sores on their skin. The diagnosis they were given was juvenile rheumatoid arthritis. They could not get around without crutches. Soon, her husband also developed the same illness.

Far from being 'mad', as the official version had it, Polly was a remarkably intelligent woman. She started playing Sherlock Holmes, or rather, Miss Marple. Her personal investigation, initiated in 1971, soon enabled her to identify 14 cases similar to her own, particularly in children. No longer willing to tolerate the inertia of her local doctors, in 1973, Polly picked up the telephone to alert the authorities, the Connecticut State Health Department. This would create problems for her General Practitioner, who would reproach her for what he considered an inappropriate call. Polly, a true self-taught epidemiologist, increased her case-list through systematic telephone investigations. Again and again she contacted the State Health Department, where she became known as ... 'a nutcase'. She was accused of confabulation. Why? Arthritis is neither contagious nor subject to compulsory reporting.

One evening in 1975, Polly received a call from a psychiatrist, Dr Judith Mensch, who had heard of her. This psychiatrist, another Lyme resident, was herself ill, and had been diagnosed as 'depressive' by her colleagues. Her daughter and neighbour had also fallen ill, presenting with similar symptoms. Dr Judith Mensch had also alerted the State Health Department. A physician can't be sent packing as might a 'common patient' or a 'nutcase'. It was at that point that the Connecticut State Health Department decided to place an epidemiologist, David Snydman, on the case.

Official investigation at Lyme

The strange thing from the beginning of the 'Lyme affair' was that Dr David Snydman was an Epidemic Intelligence Officer. He was trained at the Epidemic Intelligence Service of the world-renowned Centers for Disease Control and Prevention (CDC) in Atlanta, Georgia – the Federal centre for surveillance of diseases, also tasked with their prevention.

The Epidemic Intelligence Service was set up in 1951, during the Korean War, for the purpose of training scientists to research biological warfare techniques. During the Cold War against the Communists, the United States feared the use of biological warfare, which had been waged earlier by the Soviets, the Nazis and Japanese, before and during the Second World War. The service had trained many soldiers as well as civilians collaborating with the army. Experts trained by the Epidemic Intelligence Service were then assigned to operational army medical units, research institutes, the media, or intelligence services.

Dr Snydman started his mission by telephoning Dr Judith Mensch, the psychiatrist who was ill, followed by a call to the now-notorious Polly Murray. He proceeded to consult the list and clinical records of patients compiled by Polly (35 of them, all of whom had waived their right to anonymity) and visited Old Lyme to investigate. Upon returning to his office, Dr Snydman declared: 'There is a hell of a lot of arthritis out there'. Snydman contacted – as if by chance – a medical colleague who had earlier trained with him at the Epidemic Intelligence Service, Dr Allen Caruthers Steere. Dr Steere was now a practising rheumatologist at Yale University. Our two biological warfare specialists observed that the incidence of arthritis was 100 times higher in Lyme than in the rest of the United States. The recent cases, occurring in localised pockets, started mostly in the summer months. Polly had made an appointment with a physician at Yale University, but she was asked to see Dr Steere instead. The latter received her very kindly in 1975, gained her trust, and began his history-taking.

Dr Allen Caruthers Steere, a young rheumatologist, investigated, then declared he was seeing a new rheumatic disease whilst refuting an infectious hypothesis of any kind. However, in time, it emerged that a large proportion of patients had suffered a tick bite and/or a round, red lesion (erythema) on the skin, often at the bite site. This erythema, varying in size, could reach several centimetres or more and typically spread outwards, with a lighter centre, the active edge remaining red. This is the famous 'bull's eye rash' described in earlier chapters, characteristic of Lyme disease called, erythema migrans.

There had been reports of this type of rash in Europe since the early twentieth century, but no-one had been willing to establish the connection. True, a few contemporary American scientists did suspect an infectious origin to this disease, which at the time was known as 'Lyme arthritis' because of the frequency and severity of the joint symptoms attending it. Allen Steere, however, a rheumatologist himself, did not, or *would not* pay attention to the interconnection of non-rheumatological symptoms integral to the disease. Nor did he trouble to seek local dermatologists' counsel. He vehemently denied any connection between musculo-skeletal symptoms and erythema migrans. Furthermore, he ignored, if he ever sought at all, the relevant medical publications, specifically earlier European research upon the subject between 1883 and 1974 – spanning almost a century. Had the denial of Lyme disease already begun?

Isolated cases of the disease probably existed in the United States before the Old Lyme epidemic. In American scientific literature, the first case of migrating redness appeared in a manual in 1956. Later, the first detailed American report of erythema migrans, in 1970, was drawn up by Rudolph Scrimenti. Scrimenti, a dermatologist who was familiar with the European descriptions of erythema migrans by the Swedish doctor Hellerström, applied the diagnosis to a huntsman from Wisconsin who also complained of joint and neurological problems. Scrimenti linked this disease to the multiple tick bites the man had sustained. Today, Wisconsin, to the west of the Great Lakes, is one of the most stricken states in America, in incidence only fractionally below that of the north-east of the United States.

Steere persisted in ignoring the experience of the 'Old World', while other American doctors brought relief or healing to patients through the use of antibiotics.

For ages, Steere busied himself in defence of the autoimmune origin of the disease, but at length the epidemic nature of the cases was so obvious that it forced him to change course. His thesis had lost all scientific credibility, and Steere had to accept the disease's infectious origins – the very possibility he had ignored for so long. Yet shortly before that point, in 1974, Weber, in Germany, had reported once again in the medical literature the efficacy of antibiotic treatment for erythema migrans. In 1976, Steere, taking credit for Polly Murray's work, at last suggested that his 'Lyme's arthritis' probably had an infectious cause, but now affirmed that the latter was a viral agent, which did not respond to antibiotics. Polly the patient tried in vain to convince Steere that the non-rheumatic symptoms of the disease stemmed from the same source and that he should test the efficacy of antibiotics. It is a terrible thing when patients know better than doctors and terrible when doctors ignore Sir William Osler's admonishment: 'Listen to patients; occasionally they are right!'

Steere then met army physician Major William Mast from the Medical Corps of the US Army Reserve, a doctor who had taken the trouble to acquaint himself with the relevant scientific literature, and had, since 1975, successfully treated 10 cases of erythema migrans with antibiotics, following the lead given by European research. In 1977, Mast, in collaboration with Burrows, proceeded to chronicle the efficacy of the antibiotic erythromycin in the *Journal of the American Medical Association*.

In 1970, a paediatrician from Hamden, Connecticut, Dr Charles Ray, had noticed by chance the efficacy of antibiotics on a first patient. Knowing little about the disease or its origin, he had thus treated many cases of 'Lyme arthritis' with antibiotics. He further observed that many patients suffered a relapse, which required an extended course of antibiotics. Nor had it escaped him that the disease often assumed a chronic course. It is interesting to relate that, in 2007, the American health authorities descended upon this forward-thinking physician to bar him from practising medicine because of his views on chronic Lyme and relevant treatments. In hindsight, one could say that such persecution was to become the norm in the realm of Lyme disease. Why? Of that, more later.

Chapter 5

1977–1979: 'arthritis' is promoted to the rank of 'disease'

In 1977, what a turnaround – Steere eventually took into account the relevant European reports and accepted the connection between erythema migrans and arthritis. He published an article on this subject in the *Annals of Internal Medicine*, seeking to pass off this thesis as his own, personal discovery.[214] In the article, Steere described the disease's neurological and cardiac complications but, true to form, asserted that 'his' disease bore no connection to the disease described in Europe.

It is a matter of record that, from his earliest involvement in Old Lyme, Steere emphasised that the American disease caused far more joint symptoms than that in classical European descriptions. He systematically minimised other symptoms, especially neurological, in spite of their extent being widely observed and reported in the United States. At heart, Steere appeared to be gripped by the wish that this disease must be an exclusively rheumatological problem.

In 1979, unable to remain credible in the face of facts, he finally conceded that Lyme patients did not suffer from joint and skin problems alone, but also experienced neurological and cardiac symptoms – no different from those in Europe. The name 'Lyme arthritis' was then officially changed to 'Lyme disease'. Polly was right. Despite a quarter of a century of publications showing the efficacy of antibiotics against the disease, Steere for decades stuck to his line that antibiotics were ineffective, and – die-hard rheumatologist that he was – for years persisted in advocating treatment by aspirin, anti-inflammatory agents and/or cortisone. Yet his American colleague Scrimenti, several years earlier, had written that the cause of erythema migrans was a tick-borne bacterium in the treatment of which penicillin was effective. Scrimenti's only recompense had been sneers from his peers.

It wasn't until 1980 that formal trials were initiated in the United States to ascertain the efficacy of antibiotics. The historical overview given above demonstrates that Lyme disease, or closely related maladies, have struck humankind since time immemorial. Despite descriptions of the condition from the end of the nineteenth century, Lyme disease remained unacknowledged and undiagnosed in the United States until the 1970s.

A further twist in this tale: a sudden spike in incidence of the disease, of unprecedented amplitude, occurred in the 1970s, leading to a conspicuous surge in the number of cases. Where was the spike's epicentre? At a specific and precise location on the globe, focused upon yet again, Old Lyme, about 150 kilometres from New York, directly opposite Plum Island – a military research facility on the north-eastern tip of Long Island.

Willy Burgdorfer, discoverer of the tick-borne bacterium responsible for Lyme disease

As explained above, it was many years before the American scientific community recognised that a bacterium was the cause of Lyme disease. Years wasted, and without hope for patients. As we saw in earlier chapters, the organism is a spirochete of the *Borrelia* family, named *Borrelia burgdorferi* in homage to its discoverer, Willy Burgdorfer. As I have outlined and will say more about later, it has subsequently been discovered that this disease can be caused by species of *Borrelia* other than *Borrelia burgdorferi.*

Who was Willy Burgdorfer, the discoverer? Microbiologist Wilhelm ('Willy') Burgdorfer, was of Swiss-German origin, and was born in Basel. He studied at the university in his hometown, and after that at the Swiss Institute for Tropical Diseases. He then gained a doctorate in zoology, parasitology and bacteriology. He further studied entomology (insects and arachnids). The subject of his PhD thesis was the lifecycle of the spirochete responsible for an endemic relapsing fever in East Africa, *Borrelia duttonii*, transmitted by the soft tick *Ornithodoros moubata*.

He also researched the factors at play in the transmission of a tick's injection of *Borrelia* ('inoculum') into a host animal following a bite and blood-meal. He also contributed to the investigation into Q fever cases in various regions of Switzerland. Q fever is an infectious disease caused by *Coxiella burnetii*, a bacterium liable to assume a chronic course and damage a patient's heart valves. Q fever probably arrived in Europe with contaminated sheep carried on boats by the Australian army to help Europe against the Germans.

Later, *Coxiella burnetii* was used as a biological weapon. Human studies were performed in 'Operation Whitecoat', a bio-defence medical research programme carried out by the United States Army at Fort Detrick, Maryland between 1954 and 1973. The programme used volunteer enlisted personnel who were nicknamed 'Whitecoats'. These volunteers, all conscientious objectors, were informed of the goals of research before providing consent to participate. The stated purpose of the research was to defend the country against biological weapons and it was believed that the Soviet Union was involved in similar activities.

From that time, Willy Burgdorfer started a collaboration with an American research team at the Rocky Mountain Laboratory (RML) in Montana, which culminated in his joining the Montana laboratory team in 1952. In 1957, he acquired American citizenship and became a permanent recruit of RML, as a medical entomologist. Work at the laboratory enabled him to expand his insights into the *Borrelia* genus of bacteria through experimental work upon another, related, genus of bacteria: *Rickettsia*. He researched a particular tick-borne disease, frequently encountered in the region, Rocky Mountain spotted fever, caused by a member of the *Rickettsia* genus. Later, the laboratory would become the reference centre of the World Health Organization for *Rickettsiae*. Willy Burgdorfer and the

French microbiologist, Didier Raoult worked together, especially on rickettsiosis and *Coxiella burnetii,* the agent of Q fever. In 1991, Willy Burgdorfer was appointed as Doctor Honoris Causa of the University of Marseille. They especially worked on a new species, *Rickettsia helvetica.*[39] Years later, the world rickettsiosis reference centre was transferred to Marseille, France, to the lab of Didier Raoult.

Willy Burgdorfer was thoroughly familiar with European research into tick-borne diseases and spirochetes, including *Borrelia*. Around 1950, he met the Swedish scientist Hellerström, from the Karolinska Institute of Stockholm, who was researching the bacterial cause of erythema migrans. Hellerström indicated to Burgdorfer that spirochetes transmitted by the *Ixodes ricinus* tick were the likely culprits and urged microbiologists and entomologists alike to seek the answer in the tick's digestive system. Burgdorfer later stressed that Hellerström's views were ignored.

Years after the onset of his 'non-infectious Lyme arthritis' epidemic, Steere officially appointed Burgdorfer to investigate a possible bacterial cause, the likelihood of which had been evident for years. Burgdorfer found the answer – in the tick's intestine. In 1982 Burgdorfer published in the prestigious journal *Science* his discovery of spirochetes in the digestive tract of *Ixodes scapularis* ticks and expressed his suspicion that this infectious agent was the cause of Lyme disease.[55] Soon after, Barbour and his laboratory colleagues succeeded in cultivating those spirochetes under special conditions. The infectious role of the spirochetes was confirmed in 1983 when they were isolated from the blood and skin of Lyme disease sufferers. In 1984, the spirochete was christened *Borrelia burgdorferi,* in acknowledgement of Willy Burgdorfer's sterling work. It is wryly amusing to note that, at the time, one of the leaders of the small group investigating the epidemic described Burgdorfer's research as 'insignificant' – a group always notable for the gift of clairvoyance!

Errors in treating Lyme disease

The revelation that Lyme was a bacterial disease which could be treated with antibiotics had barely been accepted when a small coterie of scientists at the Infectious Disease Society of America (IDSA) decreed that, by analogy with syphilis, the *Borrelia burgdorferi* bacterium could be eliminated by a short course of antibiotics. Many doctors had observed the contrary, as had many patients. A proportion of the sick – far from negligible – were not cured, or, if transiently relieved, sooner or later relapsed. From the earliest stages of this saga, eminent scientists had observed that *Borrelia* could mutate and persist in a round (i.e. non-spiral) form within human tissue, out of reach of treatment agents and the immune system alike – but it seemed to be forbidden to mention this crucial trait. Authors were disputed and their endeavours even sabotaged when attempting to publish such insights, and their work discredited. To what purpose? We shall in time return to this major aspect of the official version of the disease, which scandalously propelled many patients into seeking psychiatric help.

Lyme disease: a 'new plague' for New Yorkers

Karl Grossman is a professor of journalism at the University of New York, and a specialist in investigative journalism. Having suffered a tick bite on Long Island in May 2014, he reported about the area just outside New York City. He recounts his childhood in Queens with his family. His parents used to take him camping every year in Long Island, at Wildwood State Park (Wading River). They never encountered ticks. Later he joined the Eagle scouts and for years rambled in the countryside and camped with his friends. None was ever bitten by ticks. However, he reports that the region is now infested with ticks of all kinds, and many residents are affected by Lyme disease or other tick-borne illnesses. While the west side of Long Island is urban and integrated with New York City, the eastern part of the island has remained rural and residential, with beautiful beaches. Many New Yorkers travel there for weekends or holidays. However, some French New Yorkers have it that, in the Hamptons, a few kilometres from Plum Island, as you leave the tarmac of the parking lots and set foot on the grass, the ticks unleash their attack.

The different bacterial agents responsible for Lyme and associated diseases

As I have highlighted in earlier chapters, research has demonstrated that *Borrelia* species other than *Borrelia burgdorferi* are implicated in Lyme and related diseases. Indeed, in 1982, the German neurologist Rudy Ackermann isolated *Borrelia afzelii* and *Borrelia garinii* in sheep ticks. Both are now known for their potential to cause Lyme disease. Since then the list of *Borrelia* pathogens has continued to swell. These *Borrelia* species find hosts in numerous birds and small mammals, especially rodents and squirrels. Deer and ruminant mammals are also an important reservoir. In 1983, Burgdorfer, having returned to his native land for the occasion, isolated the *Borrelia burgdorferi* spirochete in Swiss ticks.

Willy Burgdorfer also always insisted on the possibility of transmission by ticks of other pathogens, generating associated infections, the resulting entities being called *'co-infections'*. In this, he paid tribute to French scientists Donatien and Lestoguard, who in 1935 found an intra-cellular bacterium in the blood of sick dogs. It resembled the gram-negative *Rickettsia* bacteria and they named it *Rickettsia canis*. The bacterium was later re-named *Ehrlichia canis* after the famous German microbiologist Paul Ehrlich. This disease is now known as 'ehrlichiosis'. Other agents of ehrlichiosis have since been discovered. This is a field in constant development.

Attempts at developing a vaccine

A vaccine was developed against Lyme disease specifically caused by the entity *Borrelia burgdorferi sensu stricto.* It was marketed in the United States in 1998 and given to subjects aged 15 to 70 as a course of three injections. During research trials, the vaccine yielded a 78% success rate in *primary prevention.* People living in areas at high risk for Lyme disease were naturally more inclined to seek immunisation, but, as the vaccine had not been tested on children, its administration was confined to adolescents and adults.

Subsequent developments suggested a high degree of pre-existing sub-clinical exposure in adolescents and adults receiving the vaccine – that is, these individuals were already immunologically familiar with the organism and had been infected, without knowing it. Subsequently there were many complaints and reports of Lyme disease symptoms developing in people who had had the vaccine, particularly joint pain resembling arthritis, with conspicuous swelling of their joints.

Should we be surprised that lawyers were the next port of call in seeking redress for the 'side effects' of the vaccine? It was withdrawn in 2002, and the episode greatly discouraged other attempts into immunisation-research due to the prospect of lawsuits and compensation of 'victims'. It is, however, likely that post-vaccination reactions were triggered in individuals whose immune systems had already encountered *Borrelia burgdorferi*, or other similar bacteria, and we were witnessing none other than 'Herx' exacerbations of symptoms.

Recently, a small number of pharmaceutical laboratories have resumed research into a vaccine against Lyme disease. Thus, years later, several vaccines taking into account several species of *Borrelia*, are under investigation. In 2020, these vaccination projects are ongoing, but without sufficient results as yet.

Chapter 6

Recent research developments

British and American interest in Lyme disease

I have worked on the management of chronic Lyme disease in France since 1994, and because of this expertise, I have become known on various European patient networks. I began to be invited to conferences jointly organised by patient associations and doctors involved in the management of chronic Lyme, the LLMD (Lyme-literate medical doctors). I would call them 'crypto-infectiologists' (infectiologists = infectious disease specialists) because their knowledge goes far beyond the strict Lyme disease field and extends across all the 'crypto-infections'.

In June 2010, I was invited to a meeting in London organised by the International Lyme and Associated Diseases Society (ILADS). This international society works for the recognition of chronic Lyme disease, and provides information about the poor quality of diagnostic tests and the role of co-infections as a source of disease. ILADS is committed to training doctors in the proper management of patients with chronic Lyme disease and co-infections. Needless to say, its members have often been made to look crazy or passed off as charlatans.

In London, I met some great doctors doing remarkable work with patients and all highly motivated in their battle for the recognition of chronic Lyme disease and possible co-infections.

I presented my clinical experience in detail and it warmed my heart to see that doctors from different countries shared the same experience. In Europe, the German doctors of the Borreliose Centrum of Augsburg in particular were very organised and already had a significant level of experience; there were also some English doctors who were seeing many sick people.

However, despite this positive experience, there were still clearly problems to be resolved. A young English doctor asked me to help her defend herself against the UK's National Health Service (NHS), which wanted to suspend her licence to practise because of what they perceived to be her deviant practices in the treatment of Lyme. I accepted this difficult task because international solidarity seems to me crucial in such a situation. I read the report from the British expert, an éminence grise of the European Concerted Action on Lyme Borreliosis (EUCALB), a group of experts whose role was to impose the recommendations drawn up by the American 'Lyme club' of IDSA (see page 58) on Europe.

I quickly realised that this expert was not familiar with the clinical management of chronic Lyme disease and referred to only a limited part of the published medical literature on the subject. In the end, after months of proceedings, all of the attacks against the British doctor under investigation, and her colleagues who worked in the same London hospital, were lifted. It was a great joy for me. A few years later, I wanted to refer a French patient living in London to this doctor. I learned then that, disgusted by the NHS attacks, she had preferred to emigrate to Australia.

An American doctor, Dave Martz, told his story to the conference. A few years earlier he had begun to suffer from neurological problems that had worsened over time. He had consulted the best neurologists in the United States, all of whom had diagnosed him with amyotrophic lateral sclerosis (ALS) or Charcot's disease. (Americans call it Lou Gehrig's disease.) There is no cure and his doctors advised him to get his affairs in order as he had no more than two years to live.

However, while reading a book about Lyme, he had wondered if, by chance, he might in fact have chronic Lyme disease. His neurologists strongly rejected this diagnosis. His tests for Lyme disease were negative, but by sending samples to various laboratories, an unconventional test came back positive. He was by now paralysed and in a wheelchair but thanks to this test he was able to be prescribed antibiotics. After several months of antibiotics and antiparasitic drugs, he was completely healed from 'ALS'! In 2006, he published his story with Harvey.[108] Since then he has opened a chronic Lyme clinic and treated many cases of ALS with antimicrobials. He told me he had been able to improve the condition of at least 15% of ALS patients. As with other autoimmune or degenerative diseases, antimicrobial medicines work only to a certain extent. I was aware of similar cases in France and I was able to meet two patients cured of ALS whom I had not treated myself.

Whilst talking with Dave Martz, I met the famous psychiatrist Robert Bransfield, an American pioneer in the treatment of various psychiatric illnesses with antimicrobial drugs. Bransfield treats autistic and schizophrenic people with some impressive results. These two doctors also told me about their experience in treating multiple sclerosis and Parkinson's disease with antimicrobials and achieving a marked improvement in almost 20% of cases.

Years later, in 2015, Martz, in association with Bransfield, sent me a message to congratulate me on the treatment of a paraplegic boy hospitalised in a psychiatric hospital near Lille for 'hysteria'. This story was broadcast on France 2's national news programme. An internet user had found the clip and broadcast it on the internet after giving it English subtitles. I had no idea that this boy's story was going to travel around the world in a few days and I will return to it in more detail later (page 177) because it is particularly telling and moving.

During that 2010 conference, I also met Richard Horowitz, an American who, having studied medicine in Belgium, spoke excellent French with a mixture of Belgian and American accents. We discovered that, although we did not know each other, we had a similar experience on each side of the ocean. Since that meeting, we have stayed in touch. I invited Richard to present his experience at the annual conference of the French Infectious Disease Specialists, the Journées Nationales d'Infectiologie (National Infectious Disease Days), which was held in June 2011 in Toulouse.

My French infectious disease colleagues do not believe in chronic Lyme, but they were very open-minded and accepted Richard's presentation. However, when the National Reference Centre (NRC) for Borreliosis in Strasbourg learned that Horowitz was coming to the session organised on Lyme, a storm broke out as if I had invited the devil. I thank my colleagues who found an elegant solution by moving Richard's presentation to another session devoted to controversial topics. Richard was consequently treated to a full amphitheatre rather than the small room usually devoted to Lyme disease at conventions. Richard's very clear presentation in good French did not convince the masses – far from it. However, I do know that it opened some doctors' eyes.

To return to the 2010 London meeting, a humorous English joke that I enjoyed during my stay in the British capital was being accommodated in the hotel opened near Sherlock Holmes' address in Baker Street – an invitation undoubtedly to continue my detective work in the meandering developments of Lyme...

The French resistance is organised

In the late 1990s, thanks to the internet and the appearance of new patient organisations, requests for consultations for chronic Lyme were now arriving at the hospital in Garches where I worked from everywhere in France and from Switzerland, Belgium, Poland, Great Britain and Canada. The Nymphéas, then SOS-Lyme, were the first patient associations to get organised, and we must pay tribute to them because, without any financial means, they worked tirelessly over the telephone for years to help patients in distress.

The Tiquatac site also helped many patients early on. Later, new organisations were created in France, including France Lyme in January 2008, and then Lyme Ethique (Lyme Ethics). Lyme Ethique, in particular, made politicians aware of the problem, including some mayors, senators and deputies. Around 2009, some had written to me or had come to see me in Garches to encourage me in my activities. Lyme Ethique disappeared after a few years and France Lyme has restructured itself and, thanks to the number of volunteers, has been able to professionalise its activities which include patient assistance, training of doctors and lobbying.

Then there was Lympact. Lyme sans Frontières (Lyme without Borders) appeared later, and was a very dynamic group under the leadership of Judith Albertat, when she was President. Judith, who wrote a book about her medical adventure, was a pilot at Air France and then a trainer for young pilots on steering consoles. Judith, like thousands of sick people, went through the ordeal of Lyme. Other associations were created, such as Le Relais de Lyme (Lyme Relay).

My clinic was flooded with requests. My secretary Françoise Kostas did a remarkable job of listening to the countless patients who called the clinic and referred them on to infectious disease doctors throughout France. (I had to stop seeing patients from other countries.)

My infectious disease colleagues, who had until then mostly treated patients infected with HIV or hepatitis C virus (HCV), or who were looking after people with travel-related illnesses, saw the solid ranks of 'chronic Lyme mad people' arrive at their clinics. Initially, patients could easily register because, thanks to the anti-retroviral triple therapies prescribed since 1996, HIV patients who were much better could return to a normal life and needed fewer consultations. So, initially there were a lot of appointments available. Patients often came with bulging medical records and a ton of test results that had contributed to the Social Security deficit. As soon as they were asked why they had come, they described at least 15 different symptoms. However, I have since heard from patients, some of whom had had five-hour journeys to make their appointments, that they were ejected from the consultation in less than 10 minutes with this response: 'Your blood test is negative. Your doctor had no right to get a Western blot test done. You don't have Lyme. I don't have time to waste. Goodbye'.

The doctors overwhelmed by this 'disease created by internet', saw themselves as victims of a 'cult' and very quickly organised barriers to such patients getting appointments. As I write these lines, I remember with emotion the interview with Willy Burgdorfer, discoverer of the Borrelia bacterium, who described those barriers in the United States, where doctors refused to see Lyme patients and who trained dragon-like nurses to prevent them attending clinics. The barrier that was most widespread was the blood serum antibody test barrier. The clinic secretaries and nurses were instructed to request a copy of a Lyme-positive blood test before registering someone for a consultation.

The 'Schaller affair' in France*

To get around this hurdle, patients sought out a new test, Schaller's test, offered in a private laboratory in Strasbourg. This test was found to be more sensitive than official tests and therefore more

* **Footnote:** In French, 'Schaller' is pronounced the same way as 'chaleur', heat. 'Coup de Schaller' evokes the heat stroke which occurred in France in August 2003, killing 15,000 people.

likely to give a positive result. It attracted widespread interest on the internet amongst patient groups. Many sent their blood samples to Schaller's. Patients with a positive Schaller test then had a magic password to enter consultations all over the country. Consequently, during this period, my colleagues saw, with a few exceptions, only positive Schaller patients.

Naturally, the negative cases were seen by me, as well as by two other hospital doctors in the South of France and by 'crypto-infectiologist' general practitioners. My colleagues quickly concluded that the Schaller test was deceptive, going so far as to claim that its results were 100% (that is, always) positive. This accusation was in fact totally false: this test was negative in many cases. This is called, in epidemiology, an observation bias: since these doctors were only prepared to receive patients with recognised positive test results, it was inevitable that 100% of those they saw would be positive!

An avalanche of emails propagated the idea that it was necessary to close this laboratory down as soon as possible. Viviane Schaller had to appear for trial before a Strasbourg criminal court. It was rumoured that all Schaller tests were positive in order to sell a product called TicTox, a mixture of medicinal plants. Bernard Christophe, creator of TicTox, also had to justify himself before the judges. The sad thing about this case was that no one listened to the people most affected, the sick people who simply needed to be treated.

American experts punished or discredited

When I first became involved with patients with chronic Lyme disease in 1995, I knew nothing about the 'Lyme war' in the United States. However, I gradually learned, through French patients living in the United States, that there was a real 'witch-hunt' there. Procedures were launched against the Lyme-literate medical doctors mentioned above, doctors treating chronic Lyme.

Some have had to stop working or at least cease all treatment of 'Lymed' patients. I know that some university doctors who had had the misfortune of taking an interest in chronic Lyme and who had even had the audacity to want to do research on it, were persecuted by their universities and some were expelled.

The only authorised research has been that which scrupulously follows the diktats of the IDSA expert group (see page 58). However, in 2012, one of IDSA's founding physicians, Dr Burton Waisbren, a former hospital head physician and then clinic director, with nearly 60 years of research and publication experience in immunology and infectious diseases, slammed the door on this 'club' and denounced the scandal of its Lyme disease recommendations. He looked after patients with chronic Lyme mainly between 2007 and 2011 and saw the real nature of the epidemic and the seriousness of this scourge. In an essay entitled *The Emperor's New Clothes, Chronic Lyme disease, and the Infectious Disease Society of America,*[36] he used a parallel with the Hans Christian Andersen fairytale to deride IDSA's official recommendations on Lyme disease, stressing that they are absolutely not based on evidence.

Waisbren wrote that physicians will eventually have to believe what their patients are telling them. Finally, a real doctor who listened to his patients had emerged! The paper set the limits of evidence-based medicine perfectly: doctors, he wrote, must not let themselves be 'blinded by double blinding'. This refers to randomised trials in which neither the patient nor the physician knows what treatment is being given. It is not about criticising the guarantee of objectivity that they provide, but about emphasising that they do not provide an answer to everything and that these trials must not be done to the detriment of patients who should be given all possible medical help. (I go into more detail on the problems caused by simplistic research methods in Chapter 10.) Waisbren's intention was to put a new value on the humanistic component of medicine. In the United States, some courageous doctors, including Joseph Burrascano, Sam Donta, Raphael Stricker and Richard Horowitz, treated a large number of patients and also denounced the official version of the disease.

The IDSA 'expert' group threatened but 'above the law'

Following the persecution of doctors caring for chronically ill Lyme patients, both patient associations and doctors became more organised, particularly with the founding of ILADS, whose website was created in 1999. In an article published in the *New York Times* in 2001 and accessible on the internet, David Grann described the situation.[248] He said that, since 2000, Allen Steere, the man who had written the 'official account' of the disease, had begun to fear sick people. At that time, patients had got into the habit of calling him at the hospital to reproach him for his denial of the disease and the suffering this caused them – some even threatened him.

At the time, most doctors followed Steere's recommendations, and due to this, medical insurance companies did not have to reimburse antibiotic treatments. When he appeared in public, patients would carry placards saying: 'How many more of us are you going to kill?' 'or 'Steer clear of Steere'. Patients described Steere as the devil, worse than the spirochetes responsible for the disease. Early threats turned into death threats by angry and abandoned patients.

Years later, in 2017, we observed the same phenomenon in France, but more attenuated, with a patient association called 'Le Droit de Guérir' which means 'The right to heal'. This group verbally attacked opinion leaders who were against chronic Lyme, using very strong language. In August 1993, under pressure, the US Senate's Labor and Human Resources Committee, led by Senator Ted Kennedy, required Steere to discuss his findings with other experts in the field. When Steere arrived, the access corridor was swarming with people. Those present wore green ribbons as a sign of their solidarity with Lyme patients.

The committee heard not only from Steere but also from a young doctor from Long Island, Joseph Burrascano, who said he had treated over a thousand Lyme patients and written protocols of care in three languages. He denounced the fact that many researchers (without mentioning Steere, who was present), deliberately played down the severity of the disease. He also stated that several authoritative researchers and physicians had unfortunately behaved in an unscientific and unethical manner. He said, 'They adhere to outdated points of view, serving their own interests, and seek to discredit every expert who has an opinion different from their own'.

A young man in a wheelchair, deaf from Lyme disease, told the audience: 'We can no longer think, we can no longer sleep', and called on Burrascano for help: 'We need you'. Steere, amazed and embarrassed, explained that this was the first time in his career that he had ever seen a Lyme patient with this type of persistent symptom, and then explained that, in any case, all these chronic Lyme diagnoses were diagnostic errors. The audience started yelling at him. He kept telling anyone who would listen that there was no controversy in the scientific community. Under constant attack, Steere began to live in seclusion under high protection. He was afraid for his life.

The experts who enforced the Lyme law around Steere then became keen to bring all diagnostic and treatment practices under their control. They pushed the State Medical Boards to investigate dissident doctors and if possible, persecute them. Joseph Burrascano had been designated as the enemy to be shot for talking too much in the Senate. Steere called him: 'the main force leading to the over-diagnosis and over-treatment of disease'. Burrascano was under investigation for months.

I remember that at that time I was treating a French woman with chronic Lyme during her stays in France; the woman worked in diplomatic circles in the United States. She was usually treated by Burrascano and told me about this witch hunt. I prayed it would never happen in France. Burrascano went broke defending himself. He had to report on his practices to the New York State Office of Professional Medical Conduct, a sort of disciplinary board of the Medical Council. A crowd of his patients and supporters filled the corridors of New York State Capitol and took turns to call on politicians to stop these official attacks. Some patients were in wheelchairs, others stood painfully with the aid of walking sticks to support their doctor. A journalist quoted a letter written by a patient of Burrascano's: 'I think of Allen Steere as the antichrist. I owe all that's left of my life to Dr Burrascano'.

The board, after studying all the complaints in detail, finally concluded that 'there was no basis for disciplinary action'.

Other doctors were prosecuted in the United States. Many were denounced at the Medical Boards, sometimes by anonymous letter, often with false accusations or false complaints from patients. Some doctors had to stop working. Many went broke due to legal fees for their defence. Many could no longer work because they had to spend all their time providing huge amounts of information about their patients in endless administrative procedures. Some doctors even killed themselves. Fortunately, thanks to the fight led by ILADS doctors and the support of courageous politicians, this period seems to be over, notably thanks to the passing of new laws recognising the existence of chronic Lyme disease (see the final section of the book – page 291). The first Bill was passed in Virginia in January 2013, followed by Vermont in March 2014 and New York State in January 2015.

The Connecticut Attorney General, Richard Blumenthal, alerted by patient associations about the practices of the IDSA Lyme clique, launched an antitrust investigation into the decision-making process that had led to the US recommendations on Lyme disease in 2006. The investigation revealed that the IDSA expert group was full of conflicts of interest with health insurance companies, reagent manufacturers and vaccine manufacturers. This was the first antitrust investigation in history to address medical recommendations.

As Lorraine Johnson and Dr Raphael Stricker pointed out in a 2009 publication,[118] the Attorney General warned IDSA to review its recommendations, due to a flawed development process. Lorraine Johnson is the Chief executive officer of LymeDisease.org, which launched the first American national Lyme disease patient-driven registry and research platform. Raphael Stricker is a US physician and specialist in Lyme disease. Despite this judgement, the recommendations have not been changed by so much as a comma. The IDSA clique really seems to be above the law. As Paul Auwaerter (see page 62), an IDSA leader, pointed out in 2011 as the first author of the controversial article about Lyme disease antiscience,[30] the IDSA group argued that a federal judge ruled that the professional recommendations were medical and not legal, and simply asked for guidance from the experts. Thus the judicial process ended. Following the judgement, IDSA assembled a group of 'independent' experts led by one of their faithful members, Paul Lantos. Lantos is a physician at Duke University who, in a 2010 publication, unequivocally stated that the IDSA guidelines were perfect and also up to date. Thus IDSA was judge and jury.[126]

The French health authorities slowly amend their recommendations

In France, from 2014 on, Social Security (public health insurance) began a similar witch hunt against Lyme-literate general practitioners on behalf of the Order of Physicians. It was sad to see this persecution taking off in France just as it was decreasing in the United States, where laws, following the 2013 Virginia Bill, were beginning to protect doctors who treated patients with chronic

Lyme. How is such blindness possible? In 2015, a pioneering French general practitioner, Philippe Bottero (see later – pages 191, 198), was summoned to a disciplinary council of the Order of Physicians. I was filled with bitterness when I learned that this pioneering doctor had been banned from practising medicine when he had cured many autistic children and schizophrenic patients.

Other doctors were also threatened, and, at the beginning of 2016, I knew many general practitioners who, in fear, were no longer taking care of new patients suffering from Lyme. On the ground, the situation was becoming positively tragic. The fault of these doctors? Not following the recommendations of the French Consensus Conference, which were a direct copy of the US IDSA recommendations, though by that time these had been discredited in court and removed from the US National Guidelines Clearinghouse website as obsolete in February 2016.

Since the beginning of the description of the disease in the United States, 'experts' sitting on their thrones had turned their backs on scientific evidence, despising the sick that the system was refusing to listen to. Health authorities were in a state of confusion.

First investigation into Lyme disease in France: prevention

In France, there have been two official investigations into Lyme disease, in 2008 and 2012, before the National Plan launched by the Minister of Health in 2016 on which there is more detail later (page 279). The first investigation, in 2008, came about because elected officials on all sides were increasingly being called upon by voters in their constituencies to do something about the disease. Farmers, foresters, hunters, anglers and sports leaders were all beginning to be concerned about Lyme disease for themselves and for those around them. All had for many years experienced the denial of the disease, the lack of reliable diagnostic testing and the inability to access effective treatment, with few exceptions. The president of the French Senate and some Senate members wrote to me. The complaints of elected representatives reached the office of Roselyne Bachelot, then Minister of Health. The Director General for Health (DGS) called me at the time to ask for my opinion as President of the communicable diseases commission of the HCSP.

As I was well aware of the enormous controversies over diagnosis and treatment and had no solution in sight to resolve them, I advised the DGS to start by tackling information and prevention problems, which had the advantage of being consensual and did not generate any controversy. 'Hotter' topics could be addressed at a later stage. If the general public, and especially people in high-risk jobs in contact with nature, such as organisers of scout camps and sports activities, were widely informed about the danger of ticks, how to avoid and remove them safely, there would be much less contamination in France.

I recommended putting information signs at forest entrances, posters with pictures of erythema migrans in doctors' waiting rooms, in pharmacies and on the premises of professional and sports associations. It is not a bad thing to remind pharmacists and general practitioners that a red spot after a walk in the forest is not an 'eczema patch' but probably an erythema migrans, requiring a suitable antibiotic treatment immediately, without a blood test and at a sufficient dose (i.e. 4 grammes per day of amoxicillin or 200 milligrammes per day of doxycycline for an adult) for at least two weeks, more in some cases.

Unfortunately, many doctors at that time didn't even know the name of the disease. They asked: 'What is *Lime* disease?' They thought it was a very rare disease that was pretty much only seen in the United States. Meanwhile, the systematic antibiotic treatment of erythema migrans had been recommended by IDSA and the French Consensus Conference. For once we were all in agreement. Consequently, in December 2008, the Director General for Health referred information and prevention aspects to the High Council for Public Health (HCSP).

I formed a working group and invited the National Reference Centre (CNR) for Borreliosis in Strasbourg and a representative of the Mutualité Sociale Agricole (MSA), the health insurance for countrymen to join it. This group drafted recommendations inspired by the work of the MSA that had already worked on the subject of prevention. This report was posted on the HCSP website. I had asked the DGS to commission the National Institute for Prevention and Health Education (INPES), now included in the National Public Health Agency (Santé Publique France) to carry out an information campaign aimed at the general public and the professionals concerned.

Unfortunately, nothing was done, and only a few insiders knew that the notice was online. What a waste of high quality work that could have helped a great deal. I was told that we should not frighten people, that local elected representatives and tourist offices would think we were stressing inhabitants of rural communities and also tourists, putting them off. Yet, this process had originally been launched by local elected officials.

Fortunately, despite this official silence, knowledge of the disease and risks to health from ticks has been increasing on the ground, and individuals are beginning to take preventive measures. According to many of my patients who live in the countryside with domestic animals, the veterinary repellents that are now available for animals seem very effective. They are given orally, mixed with food at regular, spaced intervals. This way, dogs who usually pick up ticks, can roam in the forest without bringing these charming mini-beasts home. Be careful, however; humans should not take these veterinary products; we do not know their potential toxicity for us.

However, around the year 2010, in the total absence of public or professional information, patients with chronic Lyme disease remained abandoned. The more numerous and better organised patient associations had begun to provide more information to the country's politicians and to alert the health authorities at the highest level, but lack of understanding on the part of most politicians was great. The majority of public health decision-makers bought the official thesis of the National Reference Centre for Borreliosis (NRC) in Strasbourg, that there was no Lyme problem in France since it was a 'fake' disease and a 'false' epidemic orchestrated by the internet.

The 'Institut de Veille Sanitaire' (Institute of Sanitary Surveillance), the French equivalent of the US's CDC (though much smaller), and now included in Santé Publique France (Public Health France), the administrative head of reference centres in France, had always followed the advice of the NRC. In order to understand the reality and complexity of the problem, politicians and administrative officials needed to be immersed in the concrete reality of chronic Lyme.

Due to my statements and advocacy for the recognition of the disease, officials in decision-making structures started looking at me strangely, wondering why I was leaving the beaten track. The private conversations I had with several decision-makers were always open and courteous, but that was as far as it went. Nevertheless, one day, while I was in the middle of visiting patients in my ward, I received a telephone call from a person in charge of the Directorate-General for Health reminding me that in my position as committee chairman at the HCSP I had a duty to show some reserve and that I had to stop talking about Lyme. I replied that, if this posed a problem, I could resign immediately from the HCSP, but that I would never abandon the patients and that I kept at their disposal the numerous scientific publications supporting my position. People who question my point of view have always lacked scientific arguments to contradict obvious facts; after they have heard me, I have had to deal with embarrassed silence.

Chapter 6

Second investigation into Lyme disease in France: diagnosis and treatment

The Minister of Health, Marisol Touraine, caught in the turbulent controversies around the diagnosis and treatment of Lyme disease, had the Director General for Health refer the matter to the HCSP again in July 2012. By contrast with the consensual nature of exchanges concerning information and prevention, we were now entering the hard part of the polemic and everyone was aware of my commitment. I was uncomfortable receiving the referral because I thought that, if I joined the working group as an expert, my critics might say that I had unfairly 'biased' the group and its work. I therefore decided to exclude myself from the outset to avoid any conflict of interest with the disease. The HCSP had the same reasoning with regard to the NRC for Borrelioses in Strasbourg. The patient associations would have reportedly protested that the NRC had 'biased' the group's recommendations. It was decided that the NRC and I would be heard as expert witnesses but would not be members of the group. I considered this approach to be fair and very relevant because it gave full legitimacy to the work of the working group.

The group's set up was entrusted to a recognised HCSP expert, Professor Patrick Zylberman, sociologist. I found this approach of entrusting the working group to a sociologist who was not a specialist in Lyme disease very clever because it made it possible to avoid bias. This is how Patrick Zylberman rigorously formed a multidisciplinary group, including recognised figures in microbiology, infectious diseases and veterinary medicine. In addition to hospital and university specialists, who were not very committed to the cause of chronic Lyme, he was able to integrate a general practitioner and a hospital doctor experienced in the management of chronic Lyme. This working group heard from several French and even foreign experts and, for the first time, from patient associations.

As I was not participating in this work, I was worried about the conclusions they would draw. To my great and happy surprise, their report pointed to the problem of chronic unidentified tick-borne disease syndromes and acknowledged the patients as having a genuine illness. The experts looked at the blood serum antibody tests for Lyme marketed in France and were surprised to see that there were huge problems in the calibration and definition of results. Those experts found that most of the tests marketed in France were not reliable. They also stressed the possible role of co-infections – that is, infections other than *Borrelia burgdorferi.* The working group also stressed the need to seek advice from specialist doctors in the event of suspected post-tick-bite chronic disease with negative blood test results and to prescribe an empiric antibiotic treatment, as a diagnostic test, when all other causes had been ruled out.

What a step forward! Even though I did not agree with some points in the report, I vowed not to intervene in the group and to respect their conclusions. (The points with which I did not agree when the report was finalised were the recognition of the 2006 Consensus Conference, the need to maintain a two-tier blood test that would only allow a Western blot if the Elisa was positive, and maintaining the limit on positive serology tests to no more than 5% within any locality. Indeed, EUCALB recommended at that time that serology (the search for antibodies in blood serum samples) should be calibrated on healthy blood donors within each region in order never to detect more than 5% of people as positive for Lyme disease.[28])

However, I also noted with concern that at each intermediate presentation of the report during the committee meetings, the representatives of the Institut de Veille Sanitaire, acting as lawyers for the NRC, shared a list of counter-arguments to demand amendments to the text.

As I had promised myself, I did not intervene, but with great sadness I witnessed the surreal moment when the legitimacy of the 2006 Consensus Conference and the two-stage antibody test were re-established in the report, once again insisting that a patient must have a positive Elisa test before having the right to ask for a Western blot, when the report had originally suggested quite the opposite, recognising that blood tests could be falsely negative. This explains contradictions between some statements in the main text of the report and the conclusions. Unfortunately, these two points were the only ones retained by the Social Security and the Order of Physicians to convict doctors who prescribed Western blots when the ELISA was negative and who treated patients with negative blood tests.

The opinion and report were voted on by the HCSP in March 2014. In the controversial climate that raged, the DGS held back publication for months. It was not until December 2014 that the HCSP website put it online. This had a very positive effect because it made many people aware that the Lyme problem was not a war between madmen and charlatans on the one hand and very serious people on the other. Some well-known and respected experts, who were not Lyme protagonists, recognised that this disease raised some serious unresolved issues on a scientific basis. This independent HCSP report thus made it possible to change the way politicians and the media viewed Lyme disease so it was no longer thought to be an imaginary disease or a shameful psychiatric illness. With little or poor-quality published treatment data, the HCSP experts were not able to comment too strongly on treatment, and I understand their caution when it comes to that point. I fully share with them the medical community's concerns about the development of antibiotic resistance, and this subject must be an integral part of research projects on treatments for chronic Lyme disease.

American health authorities acknowledge Lyme disease as an epidemic

In the US, the dissonance between patients officially diagnosed by two–tier antibody testing as recommended by IDSA and the daily practice of many doctors was no longer tenable. According to a survey which was not published, more than half of United States doctors no longer followed IDSA recommendations but used those of ILADS. Epidemiologists from the CDC then modified the criteria for disease notification (CDC National notifiable diseases surveillance system (NNDSS): Lyme disease (*Borrelia burgdorferi*) 2011 case definition).

From then on, an American doctor had to declare a patient who had a positive Western blot test, despite a negative Elisa result, as suffering from Lyme disease. This was an important development. Meanwhile, some doctors and laboratories that have followed this diagnostic pattern are still persecuted in France in 2020.

Moreover, the CDC, knowing the limitations of the blood tests, asked doctors, in their 2011 recommendations, to declare as 'probable' Lyme disease those cases where clinical signs were characteristic or very suggestive of Lyme disease despite negative antibody tests, if other possible diagnoses had been ruled out. This was an even more important development.

In August 2013, CDC experts announced that the Lyme disease epidemic was surpassing that of HIV-AIDS and that it was becoming a frightening health problem: 'Lyme disease rates have risen 10 times higher than previously reported', from 30,000 to 300,000 cases per year. CDC experts announced those results during the 13th International Conference on Lyme Borreliosis and other Tick-Borne Diseases held in Boston, the stronghold of the IDSA Lyme 'expert' group.

Not to be put off, the IDSA 'expert' group led by Steere's successor, Gary Wormser, acknowledged the publication of the CDC results, but stated: 'these criteria are only valid for statistical purposes and it is out of the question that they are taken into account for patient diagnosis or treatment by doctors'. How on earth, since this official announcement of the CDC, has the number of cases reported each year in the United States 'decreased' to around 30,000 as if nothing had happened? Following the old way of counting, 30,000 cases were notified, while following the new way (considered as an 'estimation'), 300,000 cases were recorded. In fact, the two ways of counting cases were maintained.

Yet the spread of the disease continued to worry the American authorities. In August 2015, a paper by Kugeler in the journal *Emerging Infectious Diseases* reported that the number of counties classified as 'high incidence Lyme disease areas' had increased by more than 320% in less than 10 years in north-eastern US states (the initial birthplace of the disease) and by about 250% in the north-central states (west of the Great Lakes, especially Wisconsin).

Where are we now?

In 2020, data are available for 2018. According to the CDC website, there were 33,666 cases of Lyme disease in 2018, but the real number of probable cases is no longer mentioned at the Federal level. Information can be obtained from some states. For example, according to the CDC website, in 2016 in Connecticut, there were officially 1859 cases of Lyme disease reported but the estimated incidence was 1980 cases per 100,000.[131] In that year, there were 3,578,000 inhabitants in Connecticut, thus the estimated number of Lyme disease cases was 70,844, 38 times-higher than the official number. Independent evaluations estimate the annual number of Lyme cases in the USA to exceed 400,000 (Bay Area Lyme Foundation, Canlyme, Lyme Disease Association).

After the official revelation, in 2013, of the scale of the Lyme epidemic in the United States by the CDC, the largest epidemiology centre in the world, this step back raises many questions. Normally, this public recognition of a major public health problem would have pushed the authorities to encourage research and action. Why this code of silence on Lyme disease? And why, despite a court decision, did IDSA's recommendations still not change? As I'll explain later, in June 2019 IDSA released a draft of new Lyme Disease guidelines, quite similar to those of 2006. Who is really pulling the strings behind this group of self-proclaimed IDSA experts? And, who in Europe, behind the group of self-proclaimed EUCALB experts? As I explain later, EUCALB was replaced in 2017 by ESGBOR, but that did not change anything.

The answer to these questions is not obvious because multiple causes are involved. These range from the influence of historical scientific thinking to personal rivalries, including the possible perverse effects of institutional structures, the difficulty of accepting a new paradigm, and even the fear of exposing public finances and insurance companies to budgetary problems. Meanwhile, Lyme disease is now recognised as the most controversial disease in the history of medicine, and when new scientific data emerge, nothing changes. It is as if there is a black hole in space that swallows any new knowledge.

Chapter 7

The persecution of those at the forefront of Lyme disease research

The death of Willy Burgdorfer

In April 2014, I was lucky enough to be invited to Erfurt, Germany, for an international congress organised by the Deutsche Borreliose Gesellschaft, the German Borreliosis Society. The president, Hartmut Prautzsch, was a Professor of mathematics at the University of Karlsruhe, and the congress was organised by two doctors, Professor Karl Bechter, a psychiatrist at the University of Ulm, and Dr Oliver Nolte of Constance. I was impressed by the intelligence and scientific culture of the organisers. Karl surprised me with his immense medical learning and his perfect knowledge of internal medicine and neurology. He had read the treatises of former German researchers on the physiology of the nervous system. A real psychiatrist! I was pleased to meet colleagues from many European countries as well as some from America. I met doctors, some for the first time, who had all had fascinating experience with crypto-infections. In addition to clinicians, there were some top researchers. All of them were very serious and had carried out some excellent scientific work, but many complained about censorship from medical journals because they had had trouble publishing their work. I met Professor Garth Ehrlich, an American microbiologist related to the German microbiologist Paul Ehrlich, who gave his name to the *Ehrlichiae* bacteria, also transmitted by ticks (see page 94). Garth Ehrlich gave a remarkable presentation on new techniques for detecting various microbes.

I also met Eva Sapi, author of works that refer to the persistence of *Borrelia* in biofilms. Biofilms are semi-solid constructions made by microbes in our tissues and in which they hide and live away from attack. Biofilms look a little like microscopic 'Smurf houses', or corals seen in the ocean, with some openings enabling microbes but also the chemical substances they feed on to come in and out. A great variety of different microbes can coexist in biofilms, a real gathering of all kinds, made up of the criminal gangs of the microbe world. Inside, one might think of being in a beehive or a bottled city. We all have biofilms in our intestines, in our arteries, everywhere...

In Germany, the situation is not always rosy for Lyme patients, but it is one of the few countries in Europe, along with some in Eastern Europe, where doctors are free to diagnose and treat chronic Lyme disease and co-infections. Yet German official and academic recommendations are the same as in all other countries and follow the dictat of IDSA to the letter. But Germany has the advantage of being a highly decentralised federal country, and no one persecutes doctors. A German doctor can commonly request a Western blot if the Elisa antibody test is negative and not be threatened with the loss of his right to practise medicine. Other very effective diagnostic techniques are frequently used, such as lymphocytic transformation tests (LTT) that effectively detect cellular immunity against *Borrelia*. This is a different form of immunity from antibody production.

These doctors are, still in 2020, free to prescribe prolonged antibiotic treatments and associated antiparasitic or fungal treatments. However, German colleagues have told me that many treatments are not reimbursed by health insurance, even for Germans. Phytotherapy (medical herb treatment) has become an essential maintenance treatment method in Germany.

French patients can only dream of this! Many go to Germany for treatment, but they have to dig deep into their own savings because care is expensive, and it is not covered by French Social Security.

During a convention break, a man on crutches approached me and congratulated me on my presentation. He was German and he was both a doctor and a sufferer from Lyme disease. He told me that he was a friend of Willy Burgdorfer's, whom he had met one day in Germany during a meeting on borreliosis. Willy had German, or rather Swiss German, as his mother tongue. The two men, both hiking enthusiasts, had become friends. The doctor assured me that I was upholding the honour of the Lyme cause worldwide, which touched me very much. He then ceremoniously gave me a photograph he had himself taken of Willy making a speech. As he handed me this picture, he took my hands and said to me: 'Herr Professor Perronne, only you can save Willy Burgdorfer!' I was more than a little taken aback, as you can imagine.

This doctor explained that Willy was sick with symptoms that had worsened over time and that he was convinced Willy had Lyme disease and needed a new medical opinion. Very worried, he told me that a defensive barrier had been built around Willy for some time, to the point that he could no longer reach him by email or telephone. He added: 'Willy is starting to lose his mind a bit and he has already been too talkative for some.' I asked this doctor why he was talking to me and not to the many American 'crypto-infectiologist' doctors in the room, especially since I was not allowed to practise medicine in the United States.

He said: 'They are too afraid of the situation around Lyme and I fear they cannot do anything'. He told me that I would not be able to contact Willy myself and that he would send him my contact details so that he could call me or send me an email. When he left me, he exhorted me: 'In any case, in Willy's name and for the sick of the world, continue your fight. You are the only one who can do it in my view because you are an academic. I know you are committed'. The same day, I asked a few American colleagues if they could do something for Willy, but I could see that it was complicated. I never received any calls or emails from Willy, but I guessed that would be the case.

A few months later, on 17 November 2014, I heard of Willy Burgdorfer's death in a hospital in Montana. Officially, he died of Parkinson's disease. I still have his picture, the one his hiking friend gave me. I had not taken his friend's name down and I do not have his details in Germany. I took out Willy's picture at the news of his death and, contemplating it, asked myself: 'What did he want to tell me?' But of course the picture didn't talk, and I felt the bitter taste of a missed opportunity. After his death, I saw an explosion of gratitude conveyed by patients all over the world. It was then that I became aware that, unlike all the other 'discoverers' of Lyme disease, Burgdorfer had understood the reality of the chronic form of the disease from the beginning of the epidemic. He had acknowledged sick people's suffering.

I then discovered an interview he had given during the shooting of a documentary film about Lyme, *Under Our Skin*, made in 2007 at his home in Montana, where he had retired in 1986. I learned that Andy Wilson, leading a small team of journalists, was forbidden to interview Lyme researchers by the NIH (National Institute of Health). At the beginning of Burgdorfer's interview, Andy Wilson was surprised to see a high-ranking NIH researcher arrive at his host's house, who told him that he had been asked to supervise Willy's interview at a much higher level. The 'supervisor' justified his mission as follows: 'There are things Willy must not tell you!'

Burgdorfer shared his experience on the *Borreliae* responsible for relapsing fevers he had studied in Switzerland and, on the ground, in the Belgian Congo and in Kenya. He recalled that Dr

Livingstone, the famous British explorer and Scottish missionary, had caught a disease he called 'tick fever' – at least one illness baptised by a missionary!

Burgdorfer, in the interview that followed, as the discoverer of the Lyme disease bacterium, explained the link he saw between Lyme disease and relapsing fevers. When I heard this, I smiled as I remembered the reaction of one of the reviewers of a paper I had written for a major medical journal, who had accused me of making a stupid connection... between Lyme and relapsing fevers. As it happens, the now 'fashionable', recently discovered Borrelia, *Borrelia miyamotoi* (see page 45), can cause either Lyme disease or relapsing fever. (As mentioned previously, in 2020 we published a large series of cases of infection with *Borrelia miyamotoi* in humans with chronic symptoms.[4])

Burgdorfer insisted that the bacterium was very difficult to detect, except by removing a piece of brain or some other deep tissues that are not easily accessible. He said that chronic Lyme existed without a shadow of a doubt and that he had encountered it. He pointed out that *Borreliae* could adapt perfectly to survive in the tissues of the body and emerge up to 20 years later, thus reactivating symptoms characteristic of the disease.

Willy Burgdorfer said it all in a few sentences. Impressive! When the journalist came to the question of IDSA's official recommendations and the Lyme controversy, Willy said it was 'a shameful affair'. He indicated that the reason was political, but without saying anything more. He lamented that money had been going 'for 30 years to those who always produce the same thing, which is, nothing!'

Refining his thinking on this point, he added: 'The blood serum antibody technique must be thoroughly reviewed by people who do not write their results before doing the research.' Did he have the calibration problem (see page 37) in mind that keeps Lyme a 'rare' disease? 'Most doctors manage not to see patients with chronic Lyme disease by having their nurse get rid of them'. He was outraged by the fact that doctors did not even dare to say to their patients: 'I know nothing about Lyme disease'.

The journalist asked him what he thought about the connection between Lyme disease and some neurodegenerative diseases, such as Alzheimer's and Parkinson's? He said he thought that further research was required on the subject because many doctors in the field believed there was such a connection. I couldn't help but be moved when he spoke about this subject, as he died of Parkinson's disease. After the interview ended, when the camera was off, he said to the journalist, with a grin: 'I couldn't tell you everything!'

After I saw that interview, I began to understand what Willy Burgdorfer's German friend had implicitly been trying to tell me. Until then, like many people, I had approached Lyme disease and related diseases from a purely medical and scientific point of view, without suspecting any other underlying issues.

My trip to Norway

In 2014, at the end of May, I was invited to make a presentation in Oslo in Norway, to an international scientific meeting organised by NorVect, a Nordic association supporting victims of vector-borne diseases. The guest list included many excellent chronic Lyme disease experts from a variety of countries. This meeting, like the one held in Germany, brought together patients, doctors and researchers. Initially, the organisers told me that the meeting would be supported and hosted by the Norwegian Ministry of Health. I was delighted to hear this, but a few weeks before the meeting, the organisers informed me that the Ministry had suddenly withdrawn its support. I understood then that censorship also occurring in Norway.

I learned that the organisers were two brave young women who had become ill as teenagers and were in wheelchairs. They had no access to any treatment because the Norwegian authorities had banned all 'crypto-infectiologist' doctors who looked after chronic Lyme and had closed all the laboratories that did not follow IDSA recommendations to the letter. This was how I discovered that the situation in the Nordic countries was even worse than in the rest of Europe and North America. The only solution put forward by Norwegian doctors to these women was to let them die slowly in their wheelchairs.

The only chance of salvation was to go abroad for treatment, which was very expensive, since it could not be reimbursed by health insurance or social security. Thanks to their parents who drew on their savings, these young women were treated by 'crypto-infectiologists' in the United States and then in Germany. As a result of antimicrobial medicines, they had got out of their wheelchairs and were able to return to a partially normal life. They had then created NorVect to raise awareness of Lyme and related diseases and to advance research. When they learnt their meeting had been censored, they had had the drive to find other sponsors and continue with the event. Ironically, they were still supervised by a neurologist, a representative of the Ministry of Health, in charge of Lyme recommendations in Norway.

A few days before my departure for Oslo, the TV channel France 5 broadcast a remarkable report on Lyme disease and relapsing African fevers, called *Quand les Tiques Attaquent (When Ticks Attack* – an English version was released with the title *Lyme Disease: A Silent Epidemic*). This report was produced by Chantal Perrin, an exceptional journalist who had perfectly understood what was at stake. I was interviewed in this report. For the first time, I spoke in public about the calibration of antibody test results to keep positive Lyme findings artificially at 5% thereby ensuring Lyme disease remained a rare disease. I had never dared to do so before, despite the fact that I had proof and a scientific reference confirming that EUCALB imposed this limit on the whole of Europe, on the instructions of the IDSA. I had tried to mention it in scientific publications but each time it had triggered the anger of the reviewers who recited IDSA's litanies.

I had not risked mentioning it in the article I had written, and which was awaiting publication in *Frontiers in Cellular and Infection Microbiology,* for fear that this would lead to the rejection of my article. Knowing that my scientific literature review on diagnostic tests was in press, I felt freer to talk about the 5% restriction on television. That report from Chantal Perrin sent the network's ratings off the scale that night. I thought, however, that the impact of this television programme would remain Franco-French.

Chantal Perrin had also been invited to the convention in Norway. When I arrived in Oslo a few days after the film's broadcast, I was unaware that an English-language version (*Lyme Disease, a Silent Epidemic*) had been broadcast abroad. I was stunned to find out that many participants in the Norwegian congress, who came from a number of different countries, had already seen the film. Chantal Perrin and I were welcomed in an extraordinary and warm way. Many people congratulated her. Thanks to her film, the world would discover about the cover up of the 5% restriction.

In the following weeks, messages came to me from all over the world: Spain, Mexico, Australia, Poland, Canada, the United States, Great Britain. 'Where did Professor Perronne get that 5% from?' I was delighted to provide the reference to those who asked me. I saw on blogs in the United States, in Great Britain: 'Professor Perronne dropped a bombshell with his 5%!' but, on the side of the authorities in all these countries, there was no reaction, not the shadow of any denial, just deafening silence. This revelation increased people's awareness in many countries. Willy Burgdorfer had said it: 'They had decided on the result of the antibody tests before they developed them.'

When I arrived at the conference, on the pavement outside the Grand Hotel in Oslo a bright-eyed fellow was waiting. I didn't know him but it was the pathologist Dr Alan MacDonald. I had heard of him and knew his remarkable work on Lyme disease, but had never seen him (see Chapter 9 for a discussion of his achievements). Recognising me, he hugged me and said, 'You're a hero'. I told him that I was very flattered and delighted to meet him, but that I was no more a hero than he was as he had been working on chronic Lyme for longer than me and many other experts attending the conference. He looked me straight in the eye and said, 'You don't realise. You are a hero because you are the first in the history of Lyme, with your university status, your official responsibilities and your academic activities, to dare to say in public all that you have said and to say it to the whole world. In the United States, nobody, with your status, would dare. Too many people have got into trouble. Well done.' And he added in perfect French: 'Vous êtes merveilleux, vive Pasteur, vive la France!' ('You are wonderful, long live Pasteur, long live France!').

I was overwhelmed. On the one hand, I had in front of me, in flesh and blood, one of the greatest pioneers in the discovery of Lyme disease who had very quickly demonstrated, in agreement with Burgdorfer's position, that *Borrelia* persisted and that the disease was chronic. On the other hand, I knew that this man, now retired, had suffered a lot throughout his career because the IDSA clique had discredited his work from the very beginning.

I discovered at this conference that censorship was fierce in Norway, as was the organised persecution of professionals. Some patients in wheelchairs or lying on stretchers cried out at the pain of having no access to any doctor or any treatment. Many did not have large financial resources and could not afford the fares on top of the medical expenses abroad. The only answer from the doctors was that they were crazy. In this case, there is madness, but it is less with the patients than with those who should be treating them. Swedish and Finnish patients present in the room all reported the same scenario, the same ordeal. German patients were privileged because they had access to care. Chantal, who had investigated the situation in France, acknowledged with me the frightening reality in some countries – that was, hard-line failure to render assistance to people in danger!

The two young women who had organised the congress gave a brief, emotional but restrained presentation of their medical journey. Their account was harrowing. Censorship did not only affect caregivers; it was also scientific. Professor Carl Morten Laane of Bergen University had been banned from publicly presenting the results of his research on *Borrelia* under the microscope. This censorship was absolutely 'normal' because, according to the official version, *Borreliae* do not change form in order to persist. Censorship is still present in 2020. In this Kafkaesque context, this researcher was able to keep his wits about him and told the organisers that, since he was not allowed to speak, he would not open his mouth but he had prepared a short film for the participants. This video showed the changes in shape of *Borreliae* under the microscope, explaining their persistence in tissues and therefore the chronicity of the disease. As Professor Laane was not allowed to speak, he showed the images with musical extracts. He looked at the Norwegian Ministry representative with a sarcastic eye: yes, he respected censorship since he remained absolutely mute. The room burst out laughing. Fortunately, humour always overcomes stupidity.

The ministry representative, sitting next to me, was not laughing at all. When she introduced herself to me at the beginning of the congress, I saw immediately that she thought that all the attending patients were mad or hypochondriacs and that all the invited so-called international experts were eccentrics or charlatans. The meeting took place over two days, so I saw her change a little over time. It must be said that the medical and scientific quality of the presentations was remarkable. She was discovering a completely new world for herself and, even if she had to maintain her official position, she seemed puzzled. Alan MacDonald, the first in the world to link certain forms of Alzheimer's disease to Lyme disease, made a brilliant presentation. To please me, he read an extract from Louis Pasteur's writings in French. Once again, I was very touched.

I met Joseph Burrascano, who impressed me very much. This exceptional doctor, despite all the attacks he had suffered during his career, was very dignified and modest and knew how to keep a sense of humour. I discovered his enormous experience and intelligence. I was saddened to hear that he had eventually given up clinical work and devoted himself to training.

When I arrived in Oslo I learned too that a Belgian entomologist colleague was in trouble with her university. She had found too many ticks in Belgium and especially too many infected ticks. The presentation of her results had triggered an influx of requests for medical consultations for Lyme disease. Her colleagues laughed at her, calling her 'Miss Tick', or 'mystic'. This new episode, together with the whole context of censorship that I had discovered around the congress, filled me with anger and that very evening in my hotel room, I wrote a poem I decided to read the next day in public during my presentation.

I had a revolutionary spirit that night. In my head, the patients' tears, and the official IDSA recommendations broadcast *urbi et orbi* from Boston were rushing through my mind. *I knew that* the word 'tear' has two meanings in English: 'Tear' as in crying, but also 'to rip' and that another word which sounds the same in English, 'tier', means 'level'. I thought of the official blood test imposing two steps, the Elisa then, if positive, the Western blot. And then there was 'The Boston Tea Party', an historic event that triggered the beginning of the American Revolution against the English in 1773, when Bostonians who were tired of paying taxes on products imported from England, including tea, an English symbol if ever there was one, threw a boatload of tea into the sea. It made me think of all the scientific and political events that were occurring in the world under the growing pressure of the sick and bringing us closer to a Lyme world revolution.

I wrote this poem which played on all those connections under the title *The Boston Tear Party.*

Hello Mister IDSA
Mister no idea, Mister no assay.
Do you see something?
*IDSA (**I D**on't **S**ee **A**nything!)*
Is there a trick
To deny the fear of ticks?
Hello Mister IDSA
What do you say?
You say: Any test needs two tiers.
The eyes of patients are full of tears.
You say: Antiscience is a single tier.
Your guidelines, patients tear.
Doctors ask for a Western blot,
You say: it is a plot.
Hello Mister IDSA
What do you say?
You say: 'It's only psychosomatic,
Antibiotics are not automatic.'
When life is destroyed by ticks
What is your concern about ethics?
Bye bye Mister IDSA
You won't have anymore to say.
The Boston tea party
Launched the American revolution,
The Boston tear party
Will launch the global Lyme revolution.

After I had read my little satirical verse, the whole room rose en masse in thunderous applause and, for the first time in my life, I was given a standing ovation. It was very heart-warming. I would like to stress that this text was by no means an attack on IDSA as such, which is a highly respectable learned society that has been advancing knowledge in the field of infectious diseases since its creation, with a very positive and significant international impact. The message was only aimed at the IDSA expert group in charge of Lyme disease.

When I sat down next to the Norwegian Ministry neurologist, she was evidently afraid and asked me if I was not ashamed to be so flippant. I told her that the priority, and therefore her priority, was to recognise the suffering of the sick.

The congress ended with an exciting round-table discussion between experts and patients. The Ministry neurologist was very uncomfortable because some patients were starting to call her out, condemning the total lack of care in the country. Very embarrassed, she quickly pretended that she had to leave so as not to miss her bus. Five minutes later, one of her colleagues present in the room, fearing that questions would turn to her, also said that she had a bus to catch. The room laughed at this outbreak of desire to take the bus so urgently. It was well known that in Oslo there were no buses in the middle of the afternoon!

This Oslo congress, because of its scientific quality and its profoundly humane approach to the disease, had a big effect on me. It opened my eyes even more to the alarming situation of a significant number of patients around the world. These people were and still are going through hell daily, without hope. Meanwhile, the authorities in many countries are continuing to say, 'Everything is just fine.' If they were to take the official psychiatric view of the disease to its logical conclusion, faced with a pandemic of madness, they would need to clone lots of psychiatrists to cope with the situation.

At the Oslo congress, I was able to talk freely with Lyme disease pioneers from the United States. This was how I learned that, from the beginning, it had been decided that Lyme disease should remain a rare diagnosis and then, when the infectious cause could no longer be hidden, it was immediately declared, without any scientific evidence, that, even if it was infectious, all patients recovered after 15 days of penicillin, or perhaps three weeks at most in the more severe forms.

Since it had been obvious to many doctors from the beginning of the epidemic that not all patients were cured in three weeks and that there were many cases of relapse, the solution came readily from the experts: if the patients continued to complain after three weeks, it could no longer be Lyme disease – instead they quickly invented the astonishing concept of 'post-Lyme syndrome', which is a big catch-all worthy of a rubbish bin with selective sorting for chronic fatigue, fibromyalgia, hysteria, autoimmune disease, depression and perhaps Münchhausen's syndrome (a psychological condition characterised by the need to simulate an illness or injury in order to attract attention or compassion). Needless to say, this post-Lyme syndrome is not based on any scientific study. The problem for the designers of this phantom syndrome is that all the scientific data show the persistence of *Borrelia*, but in this context it is easy to understand why it is so difficult to publish on chronic Lyme.

In contrast, the IDSA Lyme group, led by Gary Wormser, was still allowed to publish a woefully methodologically poor article in the journal *Clinical Infectious Diseases* in 2015 (Wormser GP et al. *Clinical Infectious Diseases* 2015) aimed at persuading readers that the quality of life of patients with chronic Lyme was the same as that of average Americans.[242] The authors did not define the patient population studied and we do not know how severe their disease was, nor its signs and symptoms; we have no idea what the treatments received were nor their duration. I was associate editor of an international medical journal and, if I had received a manuscript of this kind, I would have refused it and would not even have sent it to experts for review, in order to spare them from wasting their time. It was the type of publication that can be shown to students as an example of 'how not to write an article'. It was very surprising that a text of this poor quality could be accepted by a major international journal.

Chantal Perrin's film meanwhile has enjoyed, and continues to enjoy, unprecedented success around the world. Some American experts have even called it 'the best film ever shot on Lyme disease'. Judith Albertat, the former Air France pilot who wrote a book about her medical adventure (see page 320), has become a world star. Now that her health has improved, she has started flying small tourist planes again and we see her in Perrin's film, thin, pushing her small plane before taking off. The film, licensed for distribution around the world, has been shown on a loop in some countries. Only Sweden, which is subject to a censorship regime similar to Norway's, has raised issues. Swedish television finally received permission to broadcast the film on condition that it be accompanied by a warning banner 'informing' the Swedes that what was shown in the film concerned France only and that, on a scientific level, chronic Lyme disease did not exist. It is reminiscent of wartime censorship. This was all the more distressing as Swedish doctors had been pioneers in describing Lyme disease at the very beginning of the twentieth century.

On my return from Oslo, my article on the review of the diagnostic aspects of Lyme disease was published in *Frontiers in Cellular and Infection Microbiology.*[17] I was surprised to see on the journal's website that this article, in the space of two weeks, had become the third most read article in the journal's history. Admittedly this journal was not very old, but this illustrates the enormous interest of physicians and researchers regarding access to objective data beyond censorship.

A military conspiracy theory about Lyme disease

Without taking sides on a hypothesis which goes beyond the field of medicine, it is necessary to mention investigative work that, based on geographical, historical and political data, has raised the possibility that military research on biological weapons might have been behind the origin of the first major outbreaks of Lyme disease after the Second World War. These outbreaks have, in fact, represented a new phenomenon compared to the 'background noise' made by the disease as it had existed for centuries.

Willy Burgdorfer had the honesty to distance himself from his IDSA colleagues fairly early on. We'll never know what he did before that, and he is no longer here to tell us. However, it seems unlikely that, years after the Lyme outbreak came to light, Steere's team would have belatedly asked Burgdorfer for help to search for an infectious cause that had been denied for a long time. Would Steere really have asked for Burgdorfer's help whilst Burgdorfer was peacefully spending time in the Rockies examining ticks and that when Burgdorfer arrived from Montana to join Steere and his team, he would have cut a tick in half and exclaimed with surprise: 'Well, that's funny, I can see some worm-like bacteria that remind me of the spirochetes of my youth'.

In fact, as we have seen, from the 1950s on, Burgdorfer had studied many spirochetes, including the *Borrelia* species causing relapsing fevers. He worked on different species of bacteria from various regions of the world, on different species of tick and on the experimental infection of animals, such as guinea pigs, as he published with Davis in 1954. That year was also the date of one of his articles devoted, in the tradition of Charles Nicolle, to the description of 'silent infections' that he called 'occult infections'.

Later, 10 years after his American naturalisation in 1957, Burgdorfer became a member of the Armed Forces Epidemiological Board created in 1948 and superseding the Army Epidemiological Board, itself created at the beginning of the Second World War.

We should note that the Frenchman, Marcel Baltazard, who was director of the Pasteur Institute of Tehran, a great researcher on contagious respiratory plague in Iran, was an expert consultant to this board. The board was composed of numerous themed commissions. Burgdorfer was a member from 1967 to 1972, when the Old Lyme epidemic began. In the photo of the autumn meeting of the Commission on Rickettsial Diseases held at the Walter Reed Army Institute of Research, Washington, DC, on 30 November – 1 December 1972, Willy Burgdorfer was among the 17 members present.

During the discussion that followed my intervention in the framework of the NorVect conference in Oslo, a patient surprised me with an unexpected question. He asked me if I was aware of the research on ticks and *Borrelia* led by the military since the end of the Second World War at a secret research centre near the town of Lyme on Plum Island.

Plum Island was named by the first Dutch settlers who founded New Amsterdam, which, after the British takeover, became New York. Ships sailed past this island before arriving in New York along a narrow strip of sea, Long Island Sound. The shores of the island were, apparently, covered with plum trees. This small island, shaped like a lamb chop, was a strategic site for the maritime defence of New York and was quickly put under military control. In 1869, a lighthouse was opened there and in 1897, Terry Fort was built. After the Second World War, the island was entrusted to the US Department of Agriculture to open a research centre looking at animal infections, the Plum Island Animal Disease Center (PIADC). The security of the island was entrusted to the US Department of Homeland Security (DHS).

That was the first time I had heard about this island, and I told the patient I didn't know anything about it. However,

Burgdorfer's German friend's comments came back to me and Burgdorfer's own comments during his interview – that he had not told everything. I kept those thoughts to myself.

It is true (and this is apparently public knowledge) that the Nazi veterinarian Erich Traub conducted research on vectorial diseases (those spread by ticks, fleas, lice and mosquitoes) during the Second World War, using prisoners as guinea pigs, as I mentioned earlier. He was working on developing microbiological weapons and conducting this research at the Friedrich Löffler Institute on the German island of Riems. Some highly contaminated ticks were reportedly dispersed during the war in Central and Eastern Europe.

In 1945, Traub was exfiltrated to the West, then escaped the Nuremberg Tribunal as part of Operation Paperclip, aimed at recovering German scientists. In the United States, in the years following the end of the war, he supervised research, particularly on Plum Island, 10 miles (16 kilometres) from the town of Old Lyme, the nearest mainland town across the inlet. The activities that were carried out on this island are described in the well referenced book written by American lawyer, Michael Carroll, *Lab 257 (Harper Collins* 2004). The town of Old Lyme is, meanwhile, located downstream from the migratory routes of birds and, at certain times of the year, downstream from the wind. It is also a region that is greatly affected by hurricanes, sometimes very violent ones.

It is not for me to judge Operation Paperclip, and one can understand the concern of the American authorities and army, after the end of the Second World War, about the major risk of invasion of Western Europe by Stalin, and, on their own continent, about Moscow's support for communist revolutions in Latin America. This concern was all the greater since the Russians had also recovered a large number of German scientists. We must not forget that we owe our freedom today in large part to the United States and the United States military.

Erich Traub returned to Germany a few years later to continue his research in an annex of the Friedrich Löffler Institute in Tübingen, Baden-Württemberg, West Germany, in the American occupied zone. Meanwhile, the main institute on the island of Riems where Traub had worked before had been taken over by the Soviets and ended up within communist East Germany. Tübingen is located very close to Strasbourg, on the other side of the Black Forest. Traub ran the Tübingen laboratory from 1953 to 1960. Some German doctors told me that Traub continued his studies there on infected ticks. Traub retired quietly three years later without ever being troubled about his war crimes.

The role of microbes in acute and chronic diseases has been implicitly acknowledged by humanity since time immemorial, as evidenced by historical examples, often related to microbiological warfare, long before microbes themselves were known. Thus, the Scythians, the first horsemen in history, who lived between the 10th and 6th centuries BC, taught their archers to dip the tips of their arrows in decomposing corpses to kill their wounded adversaries more quickly by causing the development of gas gangrene.

Then the catapulting of dead plague victims into besieged cities was a highly effective method of spreading epidemics. Thus, the Siege of Caffa at the edge of the Black Sea in 1347, during a war between Genoa and Venice (allied to the Tatars), was possibly an important factor in the plague pandemic, the 'Black Death' which is thought to have killed up to 60% of the European population between 1347 and 1353.

Such microbiological weapons must be handled with caution; in the case of the Black Death, the attacker was as affected by the disease as the victim. Microbes do not recognise nationalities, do not distinguish civilians from military personnel, nor pay heed to uniforms. However, in some cases, genetic susceptibility to certain infections may play a 'favourable' role for the attacker. Having found that smallpox, which killed only a third of

Europeans, killed 90% of Native Americans, the English, very pragmatically, drew the logical conclusion. Thus, in 1763, well before the discovery of the smallpox virus, the English General Jeffrey Amherst distributed smallpox-contaminated blankets to Native Americans, allies of the French in North America, in order to exterminate a large number of them. He was promoted to Marshal for this feat.

At the beginning of the First World War, the cavalry was the most important part of the army. The French and the Germans mutually exterminated large numbers of each other's war horses by spreading the bacterium *Burkholderia mallei*, responsible for 'glanders', a serious disease in horses.

During the Second World War, Japanese, Soviet and Nazi scientists conducted extensive research on human prisoners and these dictatorships used formidable microbiological weapons in China, Siberia and Eastern Europe. Alongside the 'killer' microbes, research was conducted on 'disabling' microbes, including the *Borrelia* type, which can be easily dispersed via a vector, the tick.

It is curious to observe that several experts – charged from the very beginning with investigating the Lyme epidemic and then with establishing the first national recommendations (which would in the end be imposed on the whole world) were trained in the Epidemic Intelligence Service: Allen Steere (class of 1973), David Snydman and Alan Barbour (class of 1974). Barbour is the man who developed the culture medium of *Borrelia burgdorferi*. He later directed a laboratory dedicated to microbiological warfare: the Pacific Southwest Regional Center of Excellence for Biodefense and Emerging Infectious Diseases.

Another expert, Mark Klempner, who set up a randomised, placebo-controlled study aimed at concluding that 'prolonged' (in fact only three months) antibiotic treatments were useless for Lyme disease, was involved in microbiological warfare research. The methodology of his study of the antibiotic treatment of Lyme disease was not adapted to follow the different categories of signs and symptoms from which the patients suffered and was not designed to differentiate the temporary exacerbation triggered by the antibiotic from failure. Moreover, the study was stopped prematurely by an 'independent committee' which declared that, in any case, it was not worth prolonging the treatment because there was no chance of seeing a result.

Fortunately, other randomised studies, independent of the IDSA Lyme clique, have shown the benefit of prolonged antibiotic treatments compared with a placebo, but these studies are disturbing to the chronic Lyme deniers, including the IDSA experts and are not included in the official recommendations. It is true that the benefit observed in these latter studies was limited in time because the duration of the treatments had also been limited.

Klempner later directed a laboratory devoted to microbiological warfare at Boston University.

It is also curious to note that Lyme disease was on the official list of potential diseases used for bioterrorism until 2005. It was on several official websites. Since then, the disease has quietly returned to civilian life.

I have been hearing about Lyme for over 30 years of my professional life and I have been treating a large number of patients with it for more than 20 years. I have myself noticed some serious dysfunction in the development of recommendations, for diagnosis as well as for research. My patients have never fitted into the boxes allocated for them, but even though I have always kept to a purely medical approach, I have gradually come to ask myself many questions:

Why is nothing changing?
Why is there censorship everywhere?
Why are these persecutions of doctors happening?
Why this constant misinformation?

Why this *code of silence*?

Are there any other issues hidden behind this?

I think back to Burgdorfer's phrase: 'It's political!'

A number of people have looked into this. I am a doctor and want to stay within my area of expertise. I prefer to let investigative journalists and historians lead the investigation.

Chapter 8

My experience with Lyme disease and other crypto-infections as a physician and researcher

Early work with Raymond Bastin and Eric Dournon

It seems useful and honest to make room in this book for a more personal chapter, retracing some major stages in my career as a doctor and researcher from the particular angle of my Lyme disease and crypto-infection experience. Understanding these diseases has been difficult and time-consuming and has had moments of setback and disappointment, as well as insights. I will show how experiences, meetings with key individuals and research on topics apparently foreign to the subject I was working on, provided new perspectives and led to significant advances.

I started my medical studies in Paris in 1972 and my hospital experience began in 1975. I had always been interested in infectious diseases and I had the chance to do an internship in a very famous department of infectious and tropical diseases, the former Claude-Bernard Hospital in Paris, under the guidance of Professor Raymond Bastin. This hospital was built as a series of small independent pavilions, with each pavilion housing a different contagious disease, so as to avoid cross-contamination. It was the 'temple' for the management of infectious diseases and contagious patients, and the only place in Paris that the German police, the Gestapo, did not enter during the Occupation (to the great joy of the resistance fighters who could hide in the underground passages of the hospital). Infection has always scared people.

In this hospital, adults as well as children and even infants were treated. Until 1988, an infectious disease doctor had to know how to treat all ages, from 7 days to 77 years and older. France's first medical intensive care unit was opened there in 1953 to prepare for a major polio epidemic that started in the Nordic countries.

During my time there, I briefly got to know Dr Eric Dournon, then senior registrar in the department of infectious and tropical diseases. I immediately got on with Eric, an excellent doctor, curious about everything, always on the lookout for the latest innovations. I would later meet him again when I came back to the Claude-Bernard Hospital, just as Professor Bastin was about to retire. Eric Dournon had the talent to combine great clinical know-how with great skill as a laboratory researcher. He quickly became passionate about three diseases newly described at the time in France: Legionnaire's disease, or 'legionellosis'; hantavirus (Korean haemorrhagic fever); and Lyme disease.

I have already mentioned that the medical and political authorities more or less abandoned research in the field of infectious diseases after the Second World War, as they were convinced that they were destined to disappear under the fourfold effect of progress in hygiene, nutrition, vaccination and antibiotics. So, when I expressed an interest in a career in infectious diseases, some of my colleagues looked at me with concern, telling me that I was crazy: was I not aware that the demolition of the Claude-Bernard Hospital was already planned and that the specialty 'infectious diseases' was condemned in the medium term?

After a moment of despondency, a small inner flame told me that life was full of infections and that I had to persevere in my calling. A few years later, my conviction was strengthened when I discovered the work of Charles Nicolle who, in his wonderful book *Le Destin des Maladies Infectieuses* (*The Fate of Infectious Diseases*) (*Lafayette Editions*, 1993), wrote that infectious diseases would always return in various forms and that they were 'the constant companions of our existence'. Infections may be apparent with periodic epidemics or pandemics, such as the Covid-19 pandemic in 2020, but they may also be hidden, the so-called crypto-infections leading to a variety of diseases.

An outbreak of Legionnaire's disease at the new Bichat Hospital

As far as the hospital demolition project was concerned, the plan was to merge the old Bichat Hospital, located in the north of Paris, with the old Claude-Bernard Hospital by building a new Bichat on the vegetable gardens behind its predecessor. This hospital was to be a tall building, with many floors, so solid and so well designed (including many two- and three-bed rooms) that germs would just have to behave. (It's true that the new building was better than the old Bichat's 40-bed wards.)

The transfer of infectious disease services from the Claude-Bernard to the Bichat was a painful one as the premises seemed totally ill-adapted to the isolation of contagious patients. In the former Claude-Bernard, there were mainly only single rooms, most of them very large, with a ceiling height of 3.5 metres. The floor was tiled with rounded baseboards to prevent dust from accumulating in the corners. There were large windows topped with smaller ones to provide ventilation. Each room had an individual bathroom with a large bathtub. Many rooms gave access to terraces in the open air. There were still pavilions dedicated to single diseases (measles, whooping cough, chicken pox, mumps, etc). A different world was waiting for us in Bichat.

When I arrived in this almost new hospital, I was horrified to see patients with contagious tuberculosis hospitalised in shared rooms with two or three beds, going down to the cafeteria in cramped lifts or queuing up in the radiology service with everybody else. Contagious patients could regularly come into contact with fragile, immunocompromised or transplant patients. As there were 15 floors, the elevator ride could take more than 10 minutes at rush hour, an ideal environment for germs when you are squeezed like sardines in a suspended box.

In the elevator, I would start dreaming about my beloved hospital with pavilions, handed over to the demolition teams. Shortly after the transfer of infectious diseases to Bichat, the transmission of a multidrug-resistant strain of tuberculosis bacillus was responsible for the deaths of several AIDS patients and the infection of a medical resident on the 13th floor. I could have been infected too as I was working on the floor below, in the department of Professor François Vachon. This 'nosocomial' epidemic (i.e. transmitted within the hospital) motivated me to participate actively in the working group set up by the Ministry of Health to develop isolation measures and, in particular the wearing of masks, by both patients with tuberculosis and the nursing staff. More than three decades later, with the coronavirus pandemic, a lot of debate has been occurring in many countries about the benefits of wearing masks.

At Claude-Bernard, the head nurses had followed after the doctors' rounds and rushed as we were coming out of each room to spray our hands with camphorated alcohol or lemon alcohol. In Bichat, the use of alcohol on hands was forbidden because experts at the time claimed that it did not kill but 'fixed' bacteria on the skin. It took many years, after the discovery of the extent of nosocomial infections, for alcoholic friction of the hands to be strongly recommended again, thanks in particular to the work of Professor Pittet in Geneva.

In the year after this episode, in 1981, an epidemic of a very serious type of pneumonia broke out among the new patients of this brand-new establishment – *Legionella pneumophila*.

Chapter 8

Legionellosis was first identified in Philadelphia in 1976 after it killed many people at an American Legion veterans' convention. The epidemic there created 182 cases, 29 of them fatal. The investigation would uncover a new bacterium in the air conditioning system, which was named *Legionella pneumophila.*

During the epidemic in the new Bichat, Eric Dournon, alerted by Professor Claude Gibert, head of the medical resuscitation service, tried to find out what had caused the outbreak. Both had made the connection with the Philadelphia incident. Dournon contacted the laboratory at the Pasteur Institute in Paris, which was supposed to deal with legionellosis. This laboratory immediately replied that this 'alleged legionellosis' was an American disease and that there were practically no cases in France. Fortunately, the doctors at Bichat decided to contact the CDC of Atlanta in the United States directly. The Americans despatched an expert to France who enabled the discovery of *Legionella pneumophila* in the hospital's hot water network. (There was another deadly legionellosis epidemic after the inauguration of the Georges Pompidou Hospital in Paris in 2000.)

During his discussions with the CDC in Atlanta on legionellosis, Eric Dournon heard about the recent discovery of Lyme disease in the United States and became passionate about the subject, even though French microbiologists claimed that it was an extremely rare disease that was not worth dealing with. Eric introduced the technique for growing *Borrelia burgdorferi* and diagnostic blood tests from the United States. I admired Eric for his great foresight, for he immediately understood the real issues of these two 'new' diseases, even if he had to pay for it by antagonising certain members of the microbiological 'establishment' and certain clinical physicians. It's never good to be right too soon!

Eric knew I was interested in his work. When he had developed his diagnostic tests, he took me to his office where he had pinned large sheets of paper on the wall which, put end to end, made a large painting. I felt like I was attending an historic event. There he had noted the main clinical information and laboratory results of all the first Lyme patients diagnosed in France. He taught me a great deal about the different clinical forms of this disease, including the most unexpected ones.

The first National Reference Centres for legionellosis and Lyme disease

Eric Dournon's experience and know-how were widely recognised and in the 1980s he was entrusted with setting up two reference laboratories for legionellosis and Lyme borreliosis, and these opened their doors under his direction, initially in the Claude-Bernard Hospital. Eric conducted basic research as well as clinical research there. Due to the demolition of the Claude-Bernard, these two reference laboratories were transferred a few years later to the new Bichat building, before being moved again to the microbiology laboratory of the Raymond-Poincaré University Hospital in Garches, where Eric Dournon was appointed Professor of Medicine in Infectious and Tropical Diseases in 1990. Eric unfortunately died prematurely in 1992. I met him at an AIDS conference in Amsterdam a few weeks before his death and we had dinner together. His disappearance was a real shock to me.

The NRC for Legionellosis then moved to Lyon, and the NRC for Lyme Borreliosis moved to the Institut Pasteur in Paris. At the Pasteur Institute, there was no specialist dedicated to *Borrelia*, and the centre was attached to the leptospira laboratory, which studied other spirochetes. After all, they're just little springs! The Pasteur Institute has never shown much enthusiasm for dealing with this disease and other borrelioses. This is why this reference centre very willingly developed collaborations with the university hospitals of Strasbourg which wanted to specialise in Lyme disease. The NRC for Borreliosis has officially been in Strasbourg since 2012.

It so happened that in 1994, I was appointed Professor of Medicine in Infectious and Tropical Diseases at Garches, taking over Eric Dournon's former department. When I arrived at the Raymond-Poincaré Hospital, Lyme patients had disappeared, as had laboratory research on the disease. No team in France had really taken up the torch from Eric.

Wissler-Fanconi syndrome – chronic Lyme?

During my two resident periods in Professor Bastin's department at the Claude-Bernard Hospital, I had regularly had to treat patients with non-specific symptomatology for which there was no specific cause and which Bastin diagnosed, without proof, as 'Wissler-Fanconi syndrome', also known as *subsepsis hyperergica.* They were patients of all ages with chronic fatigue, sometimes fever, a diffuse pain syndrome including joint pain, and even arthritis. In some cases, there could be renal or cardiac damage, particularly with recurrent pericarditis. This syndrome did not meet the diagnostic criteria for conventional autoimmune diseases.

Looking back over the years, this syndrome strangely resembled what we might now call chronic Lyme or related disease. At the time, Lyme disease, as described today, was not yet known in France, except for a few cutaneous or neuromeningeal tick syndromes described a long time before. The hypothesis of the authors who described this disease was that there was a minimal infection *('subsepsis')* responsible for a disproportionate general reaction *('hyperergica')* in the body. Bastin then persistently tried to find the site of the underlying infection, which could be a rotten tooth, chronic sinusitis, recurrent angina due to large cryptic tonsils, infected eczema, etc. He called these 'focal pathologies'. If the source was accessible by surgery, he had it removed (dental extraction, sinus puncture-drainage, tonsil ablation, etc) and completed the treatment with more or less prolonged antibiotic therapy, often associated with corticosteroids in the initial phase of care, followed by non-steroidal anti-inflammatory drugs.

The condition of these patients was transformed, with a marked improvement in symptoms, sometimes even a cure. However, it was often a chronic disease that could relapse, just like chronic Lyme. I remember that very few of Bastin's colleagues believed in this disease, which they considered a 'professor's fad'. Some thought the patients were hypochondriacs. Claude-Bernard's youngest doctors, who were starting to believe only what was published in major journals and validated in randomised studies, mocked Bastin behind his back when talking about this disease.

After the retirement of this great professor, who was an excellent clinician, almost no one dared to make a diagnosis of Wissler-Fanconi syndrome as there was no 'evidence' to rely on. The mechanism of the focal pathology is plausible, but with hindsight and as I remember Bastin's patients well, I think that at least some suffered from 'crypto-infections', including chronic Lyme.

Lyme disease and autoimmune diseases

As I mentioned earlier, autoimmune diseases, also called systemic diseases, collagenosis, or connectivitis, are inflammatory diseases of unknown mechanism, but where it is hypothesised that the body turns against itself by activating the immune system against the affected individual's own cells or tissues, instead of attacking microbes.

Shortly after my introduction to Lyme disease with Eric Dournon, I did a resident internship in the rheumatology department of Professor Marcel Francis Kahn, who was one of the best rheumatologists at the time and followed many autoimmune diseases, such as lupus and rheumatoid arthritis. Professor Kahn knew other rheumatologists and American internal medicine specialists very well, and he told me about the revolution that the discovery of Lyme disease had been for some patients in the United States. Thanks to the diagnosis of Lyme provided by blood serum antibody test, patients suffering from various autoimmune diseases had been able to get cured or significantly improved using antibiotics.

He had told me the story of a woman hospitalised for psychosis in the United States. A young doctor had mentioned Lyme disease and had ordered a Lyme blood test that was positive. This person's psychiatric illness was cured with a high-dose intravenous penicillin drip. I was fascinated by these stories and continued my reflection on the link between infections and autoimmunity. It has been shown subsequently, that *Borrelia burgdorferi*, under very specific conditions, presents small spheres called 'blebs', which bud on its surface. When the bacterium enters certain cells of the body, identical spheres can bud on the surface of the 'inhabited' cells, spheres that induce an autoimmune reaction against the human body's own infected cells. This explains the apparently autoimmune reaction.

I realised that the drugs then used for autoimmune diseases were either anti-inflammatory drugs, including cortisone, or immunosuppressants similar to anticancer chemotherapy, or drugs with antimicrobial properties: sulphones such as dapsone (antibacterial, antileprotic, antimycobacterial and antiparasitic), sulphonamides, griseofulvin (fungicide), hydroxychloroquine (antiparasitic), clofazimine (antileprotic, anti-tuberculous and effective against atypical mycobacteria), etc.

Some forms of Wegener's disease, a severe autoimmune condition, improve with cotrimoxazole, a mixture of two molecules comprising a sulphonamide. More recently (I'm making a jump to 2015), haematologists found by chance that patients suffering from idiopathic (meaning 'of unknow cause') thrombocytopenic purpura (a disease with platelet abnormalities in the blood, responsible for clotting problems), who often showed clinical improvement following administration of dapsone, were likely to benefit with an equally encouraging effect from an antimicrobial treatment prescribed for stomach ulcer – a mixture of bismuth subcitrate potassium, metronidazole and tetracycline hydrochloride (Pylera®). The two antibiotics this contains are very active against spirochetes. It is the latest antimicrobial treatment for *Helicobacter pylori,* the bacterium responsible for stomach and duodenal ulcers. What's the connection with platelets? It is not known at this time.

Many colleagues have told me disturbing stories about the link between antibiotics and a number of serious diseases. I know from a microbiologist researcher at the Pasteur Institute that a famous Parisian immunologist had, in the late 1980s, asked him to analyse lymph nodes from patients with myeloma, a malignant disease of bone marrow that causes immunological abnormalities. The doctor had found that some myeloma patients had significantly improved or were cured following treatment with doxycycline, an antibiotic active against intracellular bacteria. However, this researcher admitted to me that he had found nothing at the time.

In addition, many autoimmune and/or inflammatory reactions are triggered by certain antimicrobial drugs, including antibiotics, as if the antibiotic prescribed for something else was causing an exacerbation of a latent chronic disease that had gone unnoticed. It is not by chance that some antibiotics can trigger inflammatory meningitis (called 'aseptic' because no germ can be found) or pericarditis. It is enough for the nervous system or the heart to be 'inhabited' by intruders to trigger an exacerbation reaction when silent microbes are destroyed. I had confirmation years later when I realised that these, sometimes spectacular, supposed side effects could diminish and disappear despite the continuation of the drug.

Chapter 8

The years of AIDS, mycobacteria and viral hepatitis

During my work as senior registrar in infectious diseases at the Claude-Bernard Hospital in the department of Professor Jean-Louis Vildé, commencing in 1985, I saw some typical cases of Lyme disease, but I never asked myself too many questions about this disease at that time. The major concern of infectious disease specialists at the time was the huge HIV-AIDS epidemic that had been raging for a very short time. This explosion of AIDS across the world showed our health authorities that infectious diseases were certainly not going to disappear.

When I arrived at the Raymond-Poincaré Hospital in Garches in 1994, I opened a new infectious and tropical diseases department based on the unit previously run by Eric Dournon. After a few years spent at the 'factory' in Bichat, I was pleased to find again a pavilion-style hospital on a human scale, with a warm atmosphere.

As I had been deputy director of the national reference centre for tuberculosis and mycobacteria at the Pasteur Institute of Paris since January 1993, the main focus of my work continued to be mycobacteria. (Mycobacteria are a class of very hardy bacteria responsible for tuberculosis and leprosy among other conditions.) Most of the patients hospitalised at that time were AIDS patients. These AIDS years, before the effective antiretroviral triple therapies that emerged a few years later, were terrible because mortality in infectious disease services was very high. Many AIDS patients were also infected with other microbes, which caused 'opportunistic infections'. In addition to mycobacteria, I was interested in viral hepatitis viruses and in particular hepatitis C virus (HCV). I was involved in the development of new treatments for atypical mycobacteria and hepatitis C, developing national clinical research protocols with the help of the National AIDS Research Agency (ANRS): the

Curavium and Ribavic trials that helped mark a turning point in the management of these serious opportunistic infections.

How Lyme disease got into my career

Lyme disease was not my main concern when I first arrived in Garches, although the Medicines Agency had asked me to be *rapporteur* for the marketing authorisation file (MA) for Clamoxyl® (amoxicillin), for which the manufacturer's laboratory had submitted an application for official indication of this penicillin in the various forms of Lyme disease.

This allowed me to immerse myself in all the studies published at the time and to become familiar with the bibliography of this disease. Apart from the problem of patients with symptoms but negative blood tests ('seronegative'), which were clearly described in these publications, including in the most presitigious medical journals, but whose frequency was not evaluated anywhere, Lyme disease appeared to be a simple entity, easy to diagnose and treat. How wrong I was – I found out quickly for myself that Lyme was not how it was described in the textbooks.

As Garches is located in the western suburbs of Paris, not far from large forests, I was required to manage more acute forms of Lyme disease than I had seen before in Paris. This is how, quite by chance, I noticed that some patients who had been improving following three weeks of regular antibiotic treatment then relapsed fairly quickly. I remember a lady who had been bitten by a tick on the buttock during a walk in the forest. She had been hospitalised for a fever with joint pain, severe fatigue and biological abnormalities suggestive of lupus. She had torn off the tick and broken its rostrum (biting and sucking mouth part) that had remained stuck under her skin. She had a very inflamed and painful halo around the bite site. After three weeks of antibiotics, she was cured and very happy to be better. However, four months later, she came back to see me, very worried because, for two weeks, all her symptoms had been reappearing gradually – even though she had not returned to the forest and had not been bitten again. The old tick bite on her buttock had become inflamed again at the same site and, while her biological markers had normalised at the end of treatment, all the biological abnormalities had returned, including the positivity of the lupus antibody tests.

I was very surprised but, as I had already seen rare cases of relapse in other well treated infectious diseases, I decided to treat her again, and she recovered quickly from this second episode. A few months later, she relapsed again. I talked to a few colleagues who had no explanation. I treated her again a third time and she was healed... At the fourth relapse, I didn't dare give an antibiotic again, telling myself the situation was never-ending, and I sent her to an internist. I began to think that Lyme disease was not as simple as I had read in the textbooks and that we did not understand everything.

Another case enlightened me. A man in his 50s came to see me one day for a consultation because he had read an article by Eric Dournon on Lyme disease which talked about seronegative forms. He wanted to make an appointment with Eric but had learned that he had passed away. He was very anxious and seemed very disappointed when he saw me because, as I was not known at the time as a Lyme specialist, he must have thought that, like all the doctors he had seen before, I would think he was crazy. He told me about his incredible journey. He had had a job he loved, a woman he adored and had been perfectly healthy. They had just bought a house in the countryside to renovate and, as he was very handy, he had dreamed of starting work on it. Then one fine day he felt tired and began to have pain everywhere. A whole procession of symptoms gradually came over him without his understanding what was happening. He gradually became a 'vegetable', as he himself put it, and was no longer even able to hold a hammer to bang in a nail.

He consulted many doctors who understood nothing about his condition. The tests didn't show much. He lost his job and then his wife, who had been told by the doctors that he was a lazy hypochondriac. Knowing perfectly well that an unknown evil was gnawing at him from within, he kept consulting. In 15 years, he had seen about 80 doctors and 20 psychiatrists. Unemployed, without many resources, he saved up to buy train tickets to find a specialist somewhere in France who would listen to him. The main pre-occupation of the great professors he had seen was to collect a substantial private fee. They had all sent him to a psychiatric department. He ended up getting depressed, with good reason. For years he ate whole boxes of anxiolytic or antidepressant drugs to please his doctors, but nothing relieved his symptoms.

By dint of searching, and having often been bitten by ticks, he had found himself on the trail of Lyme disease. It is amusing to note that even now it is most often the patient who thinks first of Lyme disease and that, in many cases, s/he is obliged to *force* his/her doctor to finally agree to order a Lyme antibody test. Unfortunately for this patient (but it is so for most), the test he had asked his doctor for had come back negative. So, he had no hope of accessing treatment… until he read an article by Eric Dournon explaining that seronegative Lyme existed. As I had also read several publications on seronegative Lyme, I agreed to offer him empiric treatment – that is, treatment based on symptoms. He was surprised by my answer. It was the first time in 15 years that he had been listened to, but, as he still did not fully trust me, he refused hospitalisation and told me that he was going to think about it. Then one day he called me and said: 'I'm ready!' After a month of high-dose intravenous penicillin G, he was resurrected. I couldn't believe my eyes. He had regained a young man's energy and had stopped complaining of his many symptoms.

The first patient associations for sufferers from chronic Lyme disease

One day, I received a phone call from a woman who introduced herself as the president of a Lyme patient support association. She had just created this association with her daughter Fabienne, and called it Les Nymphéas, after the famous paintings of Claude Monet, because Fabienne, who was sick, was a painter and loved the impressionists. She had loved riding and had spent hours removing ticks from her horses but she had gradually become paraplegic. She lived in Brittany and was told that Lyme disease did not exist in this region – it was present only in Alsace! I hadn't know at the time that a patient association even existed.

The president of the association thanked me for the welcome I had given to a growing number of patients. She was surprised. She then revealed to me that in France there were hundreds, even thousands, of people suffering Lyme-related martyrdom and/or disabilities who were being rejected by all doctors and who, most of the time, found themselves in psychiatry.

This woman was a saint and, though penniless, had devoted years to helping people in distress throughout France. In the light of my small experience, I had no difficulty believing her. She asked me for permission to give my contact information to the suffering patients that she knew. I gladly gave my consent. Sometime later, the handyman I had healed created the SOS-Lyme association and was also instrumental in helping countless patients by telephone. Today I pay homage to these voluntary pioneers who are heroes to me.

The influx of patients to my department at Garches

As I have mentioned in earlier chapters, I did not expect the flood of patients that would arrive from everywhere for consultations, having heard about me through various patient associations. They often arrived in an agitated state thanks to the rejection of their illness by their doctors and often by their families and colleagues too. They deposited enormous piles of documents on my desk about hundreds of investigations carried out, sometimes over several years, sometimes over decades. After a quarter of an hour of my listening to them, their agitation would die down because they understood that I believed them. This is what struck me the most and it still strikes me to hear many of these patients tell me that, since the beginning of their treatment, no doctor has really listened to their complaints.

The clinical pictures were very diverse because, as is perfectly described in the many medical publications on the subject, Lyme disease can present as anything and everything. This was the case with syphilis (also caused by a spirochete bacterium), once called the 'great imitator'. Apart from a few exceptions that I can count on the fingers of one hand, these patients were not crazy at all.

When describing the signs of a disease, a doctor distinguishes the 'signs' that are objective, and that s/he may observe, from the 'symptoms' (also called 'functional signs') of which the patient complains (pain, for example) but which the physician cannot observe or measure. The problem with chronic Lyme is that many manifestations of the disease are very often symptoms and not signs. However, medical students are generally taught that, if there are too many symptoms, 'it's not possible' and so it must all be in the patient's head.

Even though I initially had doubts about the possible psychosomatic origin of the disorders in some patients, I was quickly reassured when I realised that, as soon as they were better after a few weeks or months of treatment, all they thought about was forgetting their illness, running back to work and devoting themselves to their family. Many activist patients in the associations for that matter quickly abandoned those roles after recovering. Over time, a cohort of patients developed who were much better on treatment and who felt that they had been brought back to life after nightmarish months, years or even decades. I found that not all patients afflicted for many years with the most severe forms of the disease would recover, but many would improve markedly. To get some social or professional life back again, even part-time, was for them a considerable step forward from a life of total exclusion, often limited to spending three quarters of the day in bed and being unable to go out, even accompanied.

As I was not able to discuss Lyme with my French colleagues easily, I tried to find out what was happening abroad.

What did other doctors think?

From time to time I had some news from German, Swiss or Belgian doctors my patients had consulted before and who, each in their own corner, were finding effective therapeutic schemes. One day I heard about the situation in the United States through some French patients who lived there or who had consulted there. This is how the founder of the Tiquatac site, who helped a lot of patients, came to see me one day to tell me about her experience. This woman, of Belgian origin, could not find a doctor willing to treat her in her own country and had consulted Sam Donta in Boston, who had resurrected her with a combination of an antibiotic and an antiparasitic, hydroxychloroquine. Through another patient who lived in New York and who was being treated by Joseph Burrascano, I became aware of the lawsuits that were being brought against many doctors looking after chronic Lyme patients in the United States and that some were being threatened with disciplinary suspension.

Concerns about antibiotic resistance

It is curious to see that in spite of the extensive efforts I have made over a long period of time to explain to my fellow infectious disease doctors, the pharmaceutical industry and politicians, about the excesses of antibiotic prescriptions, I am nevertheless accused, with the treatment of Lyme, of being unaware of this major problem.

In the 1990s, I chaired working groups at the Agence du Médicament (Medicines Agency) on the proper use of antibiotics in respiratory infections and I chaired the organising committee of the Société de Pathologie Infectieuse de Langue Française, (SPILF, French Infectious Diseases Society) Consensus Conference on ear, nose and throat (ENT) infections held in Lyon in June 1996. I had been struck by the deviations in systematically treating rhinopharyngitis in children with antibiotics that were responsible for the decrease in the sensitivity of the pneumococci bacteria to penicillin and their resistance to other groups of antibiotics.

As President of the Communicable Diseases Section of the Superior Council of Public Hygiene in France, I had alerted Bernard Kouchner during his first term as Secretary of State for Health about the issues with antibiotics. At that time, the Minister informally instructed me to convene a working group to develop recommendations. I had organised the first meeting in the pavilion of the Order of Malta at the Saint-Louis Hospital in Paris, in the presence of Professor Jean-Marie Decazes. Professor Benoît Schlemmer, President of the Anti-infective Treatment Group at the Medicines Agency, and Dr Robert Cohen, a paediatrician who was very involved in the management of infections in children, were present. In 1999, Bernard Kouchner was appointed High Representative of the United Nations in Kosovo before he had time to formalise the group. Consequently, the Committee did not meet again.

Subsequently, Benoît Schlemmer, with the help of Anne-Claude Crémieux and with the support of the Ministry of Health, took up the torch and drafted a national plan to preserve the effectiveness of antibiotics with a group of experts in 2001.

Anne-Claude Crémieux would be appointed Professor of Infectious Diseases in my department in 2005.

At the same time, anti-antibiotic movements were unfortunately evolving towards extremist positions. However, and this should reassure doctors and decision-makers who do not have any experience in the management of chronic Lyme and related diseases, there are leads suggesting non-antibiotic alternatives. Recent publications, by Feng, Zhang and colleagues show that different antiparasitic and/or antifungal drugs are capable of inhibiting or killing persistent *Borreliae* in vitro (in the lab), even though they are not parasites or fungi but bacteria.[84, 85, 86, 87, 88, 89, 90] Crypto-infectiologists have known this for a long time. Persistent forms of *Borrelia* may have modified receptors making them sensitive to groups of molecules other than actual antibiotics.

It is really promising to see that anti-leprosy drugs are efficient in dealing with *Borrelia*. In an in vitro study, clofazimine, an old drug used for leprosy, tuberculosis and atypical mycobacteria, was found to be active against persistent forms of *Borrelia*. This drug is known not to produce bacterial resistance. Dapsone, another anti-leprosy agent, has been found to be very effective in treating chronic Lyme disease in humans. Richard Horowitz published the results of his excellent experience with dapsone in 2016. It is not surprising that this drug works well because dapsone is a well-adapted antibacterial for bacteria able to persist in hidden forms in our cells and organs. Hansen's bacillus or *Mycobacterium leprae*, the agent causing leprosy, is the prototype of bacteria capable of 'hiding' and persisting.

We have found that *Borrelia burgdorferi* is one of the bacteria that has an exceptional abundance of function genes, genes that provide microbes with the capacity to adapt and survive in our cells. Dapsone also has anti-parasitic properties. This broad antibacterial and antiparasitic action meant that dapsone was widely used as a preventive treatment for so-called 'opportunistic' infections in AIDS patients before the discovery of the effective HIV triple therapies. It is interesting to note that dapsone is still widely used today in certain idiopathic or autoimmune diseases that probably have a hidden infectious cause. For some chronic diseases, as for many cancers, two phases of treatment are needed: an initial 'induction phase' with intensive treatment, followed, when signs and symptoms are declining, by a less aggressive but more prolonged 'maintenance phase' of treatment, to avoid early relapse of the disease. Clinical studies with anti-leprosy drugs (clofazimine and/or dapsone) should be rapidly set up to check their potency with patients in the maintenance phase of Lyme disease treatment. Clofazimine is still available, but the Medicines Agency (ANSM) only allows its use in well-defined and proven diseases. So, Lyme patients don't have access to it. The drift of drug laws has led to a narrow administrative rigour that prevents any initiative that could be of great benefit to patients. It is unfortunate that these treatment strategies cannot be studied and are ignored as this would have no impact on bacterial resistance, and fear of antibiotic resistance is the main refrain of the fierce opposition of much of the medical community to chronic Lyme.

When I talk about antibiotic resistance here, I am not talking about Lyme disease resistance, because *Borrelia* persists inside our cells, and intracellular infections are not known to become easily resistant to antibiotics unless those bacteria can also proliferate outside the cells and cause large abscesses containing billions of bacteria. This is not the case for Lyme disease, whereas it is the case for tuberculosis for which the problem of antibiotic resistance is becoming a crucial global issue. Even when Lyme disease relapses after treatment, it is not because of antibiotic-resistant mutations; it is because bacteria escape treatment by changing their form and metabolism. An antibiotic cannot kill a sleeping bacterium.

The discussion of bacterial resistance related to chronic Lyme disease treatments focuses on the overall volume of antibiotic prescriptions that can have an ecological impact on human bacterial flora. Given the very high number of patients in each country with inflammatory or degenerative diseases, some of which are probably linked to 'crypto-infections', treatment of these patients with first-line anti-infectives upstream, thus avoiding the serious complications of these chronic diseases, would probably contribute to drastically reducing the use of second- or third-line antibiotics later on. As a matter of fact, these patients are often put on immunosuppressive treatments that cause many episodes of so-called opportunistic infections requiring repeated courses of antibiotics throughout their lives. Some infectious diseases caused by persistent microbes, such as tuberculosis, leprosy and Q fever (due to *Coxiella burnetii*), require antibiotic treatments lasting from six to 18 months. It is hard to imagine that a group of self-proclaimed experts would decide that this treatment was far too long and that one month would be enough.

Thus, one could say after stopping this short treatment, that any tuberculosis patient who is not cured and who continues to spit out his lungs and lose tens of kilos no longer has tuberculosis but is a hypochondriac with a 'post-tuberculosis syndrome' who must be sent to psychiatry! This time, psychiatrists, terrified at the idea of being contaminated, would surely believe in the infectious cause. We could also promote psychoanalysis with a protective mask! Our group of 'experts' could do the same with leprosy. During the AIDS epidemic, before effective antiretroviral triple therapies for the HIV virus, HIV-positive patients who had reduced immunity were all put on long courses of antibiotic treatment, often for several years. This daily intake of antibiotics, usually a combination based on sulphonamide, helped to reduce the appearance of the famous and fearsome 'opportunistic' infections. This preventive antibiotic treatment strategy lasting years is still recommended for some chronic immunosuppressive situations. This is justified by the 'experts' and does not attract any criticism.

Saving on antibiotics is a concern for every doctor, including 'crypto-infectiologists'. This is why non-antibiotic therapeutic approaches should be given priority whenever possible. However, pending the development of new strategies, in a few rare patients, intermittent (e.g. azithromycin for six days per month) or prolonged continuous antibiotic treatment is essential.

Meanwhile, our farm animals are flooded with tons of antibiotics, creating bacterial resistance. These resistances are easily transmitted to human bacterial flora. A few years ago, a Social Security doctor, who had worked as a general practitioner in the countryside, told me the story of a farmer who had called him because he had tonsillitis. He prescribed amoxicillin; the most effective antibiotic recommended for this disease. To his surprise the farmer angrily said he wasn't going to pay for a consultation to get an amoxicillin prescription, when he had a dozen litres in jerry cans in his barn to treat his cows!

While I was visiting a battery chicken farm where thousands of birds were crowded together, barely able to breathe because they were so tightly packed, the farmer – very proud of his installation, which was more of a factory or concentration camp – showed me how in the cages, small slides, in the shape of streamers, came down from the ceiling to deliver both food and antibiotic granules. I asked to see the bags of antibiotics. There were tens of kilos of tetracyclines and fluoroquinolones (a very effective but ecologically dreadful group of antibiotics, which are known to select resistance in bacteria very quickly). Today, urinary tract infections, particularly frequent in women, have often become resistant to fluoroquinolones.

What is curious is that farmers use antibiotics not only to treat infections, but also to encourage growth. Indeed, it has been observed throughout the world that an animal, be it a cow, a pig or or poultry, develops muscular mass much more rapidly if it eats antibiotics every day. This phenomenon is poorly explained. I think it's just the fact that all these animals have 'crypto-infections' that, untreated, slow down their growth. It is also possible that antibiotics destroy the gut bacterial flora, which has an effect on how the gut processes food. The same thing has been observed in humans. Antibiotics have not only, with vaccines, allowed an exceptional extension of the life span, but they have also allowed the children of the first 'antibiotic generations' to be taller than their parents.

In Europe, the use of antibiotics as a growth factor for animals is officially prohibited, but they are still prescribed per ton in the veterinary world, supposedly for therapeutic purposes. Unfortunately, nobody is taking action in the face of the enormous economic stakes. But a new mechanism of resistance to colistin, an old antibiotic kept as a last resort to save sick people from serious multi-drug-resistant infections, has been found in pig farms. Since this resistance mechanism is transmissible between bacteria, the antibiotic in question may soon be unusable in humans. Instead of cracking down on farms, the authorities have planned to prevent doctors from prescribing more than a week of antibiotics to humans. That is tackling the problem the wrong way round.

The use of natural medicine and its return in medical practice

Another way of strengthening treatment and reducing the risk of relapse is the use of phytotherapy – that is, herbal medicine. Needless to say, this type of treatment has never been part of my medical training. It has been the sick who have taught me everything. Indeed, the vast majority of patients with chronic Lyme disease have been rejected by the health system, except for inadequate management, and many have turned to alternative medicine. By training, I am very suspicious and doubtful about these treatments. When sick people started talking to me about them, it made me laugh and I didn't believe in them. I quickly stopped laughing when I saw some surprising results. Of course, these treatments, like antibiotics, do not work 100% for everyone, but the benefit is often significant. I have seen their effectiveness in several circumstances. Of course, medical advice should be sought as, in rare cases, herbal products may cause side effects or may have some interations with drugs.

Ginkgo biloba

I noticed by chance that some patients suffering from chronic Lyme and from memory disorders had been prescribed *Ginkgo biloba* by their doctor; this plant is reputed to be active against these disorders. I was able to observe that it occasionally caused violent worsening of symptoms in the first few days, just like an antibiotic (the Jarisch-Herxheimer's reaction or 'Herx'), but that many patients felt better afterwards. This immediately reminded me of my work in the laboratory of the National Institute of Health and Medical Research (INSERM) in the old Claude-Bernard Hospital where I helped Eric Dournon with his experimental research on guinea pig legionellosis.

While I was working with these guinea pigs, the managers of the pharmaceutical laboratory selling Tanakan® (extract of *Ginkgo biloba*) came to see the director of the INSERM unit, Jean-Jacques Pocidalo. They gave him a large scientific file, confidential to the laboratory, demonstrating the many antimicrobial properties of *Ginkgo biloba*. This exceptional plant is resistant to most infections in nature. The firm's managers wanted researchers in the unit to test Tanakan® in experimental infection models. They were hoping to develop this product in the field of infectious diseases. Pocidalo asked me to conduct some experiments. As I was working on guinea pig legionellosis, I suggested trying it on some of these animals. It worked! I was very impressed and spoke to my clinical boss who felt I had more serious research to do rather than testing plants. Pocidalo did not insist, and I did not continue this research and never published, for lack of having reproduced the experiments.

As I remembered these results with *Ginkgo,* I started to offer it to my Lyme patients, and three quarters felt a benefit. Often *Ginkgo* initially triggered several of the 'side effects' described on the usage leaflet, but then these symptoms, which are sometimes strong, disappeared, showing that they were temporary exacerbations and not side effects. I even saw a patient who did not want to take antibiotics for ecological reasons, get cured with *Ginkgo* only. Unfortunately, this product, like all the others, does not work for everyone.

A wide variety of plants can have an effect

Another time, I saw a patient who smelled very strongly of garlic. He explained to me that he had waited nine months to see me because of the demand for my time and that in the meantime he had treated himself with garlic in large doses. Asking him what dosage he had chosen (it was not to file a marketing application with the Medicines Agency!), he told me three heads of raw garlic a day. (I mean three heads and not three cloves, which is a huge amount every day.) I understood where the smell was coming from! As he was very happy with his treatment, which had almost cured him, he did not want me to prescribe another, more 'official' one.

I remembered then that I had read a laboratory article mentioning that garlic had an effect against the tuberculosis bacillus, so why not against *Borrelia*? The activity of garlic on persistent forms of *Borrelia* has since been demonstrated.[90] Similarly, when I took bacteriology-virology courses at the Pasteur Institute in 1982–1983, we were taught about the potential antimicrobial role of plants against infectious diseases. During the lecture on bubonic plague we were told about the 'Elixir of the four thieves'. The plague wreaked havoc and brought terror to the whole population. Boccaccio, the author of *The Decameron*. wrote about the 'Black Death' of the fourteenth century: 'In those days, you had lunch with your parents and friends, and dinner in the evening with your ancestors in the other world'.

During the plague epidemic which ravaged Toulouse from 1628 to 1631 and killed more than 50,000 people, four thieves were caught in the act of robbing plague victims. How did they do this without becoming ill themselves? The archives of the parliament of Toulouse record: 'Four thieves were convicted there, during the former great plague, of finding plague victims, strangling them in their beds and then robbing their houses. They were sentenced to be burned alive and, in order to soften their sentence and avoid being hanged, they divulged their secret'. The authorities, however, did not keep their word and they were hanged anyway.

The recipe must have been preserved and passed on, however, because during the plague epidemic in Marseille in 1720, other thieves were arrested in the same circumstances and handed over their protective recipe. Their lives were spared. The Marseille's authorities not only kept their word but had the intelligence to make the recipe for the elixir generally available, thereby saving many inhabitants. The thieves, thanks to their knowledge of herbalism, had concocted an explosive mixture that protected against the dreaded plague bacillus, *Yersinia pestis*, not yet known at the time. The elixir contained cider vinegar, ortigia-silica, garlic, cinnamon, cloves, lavender, mint, rosemary, common rue, clary sage, thyme, absinthe, chicory, nutmeg and camphor – only good things, except perhaps common rue, reputed to cause abortion in high doses.

There have been variations in the composition of this 'elixir' throughout history and regions. The French king Louis XV, had a famous mustard-vinegar maker, Antoine Maille, whose grocery product was said to protect against infections. Supreme recognition, the 'Elixir of the four thieves' was included in the Codex (registry of medicines) in 1748. More recently, it was not the same with TicTox (see page 103), a mixture of plants widely used for chronic Lyme disease, to the great satisfaction of patients. Its inventor was put on trial at the Strasbourg criminal court!

To come back to Lyme disease and phytotherapy, over time I have seen more and more patients treat themselves successfully with various plant extracts, including propolis and grapefruit seed extract. Propolis is a mixture of plant extracts and bee secretions whose secret recipe has been kept since time immemorial. The word 'propolis' comes from ancient Greek and refers to the 'entrance to a city'. Bees use the substance to protect against moulds and as a natural antibiotic. When a bulky animal enters the hive, the bees kill it by stinging but they are not big and strong enough to take it out of the hive. Leaving the animal to rot would destroy all the bees through the spread of putrefaction. The bees have everything planned: they surround the corpse with propolis which, therefore, does not rot. This amazing product was already used by Hippocrates in Ancient Greece to treat rheumatism, and perhaps Lyme disease patients of that time. In Egypt, it was used for embalming. Propolis was used in the Roman and then Napoleonic armies to disinfect wounds.

Among natural products, grapefruit seed extracts and melittine contained in bee venom have been studied in laboratory experiments where their effectiveness against *Borrelia* has been confirmed; this work has been the subject of scientific publications.[43, 212] Of course, bee venom is not used routinely, but it is interesting to note that in Chinese medicine, as well as in clinics in Asia, Europe and the United States, bee stings are used to treat multiple sclerosis.

The list of medicinally active plants is very long but no clinical studies have validated their use. It is almost impossible to carry out these studies because they are very expensive. Since plants cannot be patented, no phytotherapy laboratory wishes to invest because it would have no chance of obtaining a return on investment. A mixture of plants can be patented, but anyone could copy it or, to circumvent the patent by slightly changing the composition. During the Second World War, the Vichy regime in occupied France abolished the herbalist diploma in order to give pharmacists the monopoly of the delivery of medicinal plants and advice on their use. Herbalists who had already graduated were allowed to continue practising, but now they are all dead or very old. They had the same fate as home distillers.

Unfortunately, pharmacists mostly do not have much experience with phytotherapy and are not capable of providing sound advice in this area. Moreover, there are regular attempts by lobbyists to the European Union to ban trade in medicinal plants, which compete with certain industrial medicines. It is a paradox when we want to fight against the abuse of antibiotics and when we want to reduce Social Security expenditure. With years of hindsight on a very large number of patients, it is clear to me that patients who continue long-term or even lifelong phytotherapy relapse infinitely less often than others. The principle is to change the product from time to time to keep a sustained action.

Unfortunately, phytotherapy is not effective in all patients. In addition, each plant used for the first time can trigger a reaction of initially worsening symptoms, which can make the patient believe that he or she is relapsing or experiencing side effects.

The Germans are ahead in this area. I recently learned from a French colleague that German doctors at the Charité Hospital, one of Berlin's best-known hospitals, were practising phytotherapy and studying it in depth in some cases. Phytotherapy often makes people laugh; it is regularly criticised. It is particularly curious to observe this when it is sometimes recommended in practice by those who condemn it in theory. I am, in particular, thinking of a doctor at the Strasbourg University Hospital, belonging to the department which was at the origin of the legal complaint against the manufacturer of TicTox, a mixture of plants which was very popular with patients, as I have said, and which had not been the subject of any complaint on their part. This doctor declared publicly and mentioned in a presentioan, in June 2015, during a meeting organised by the NRC for Borreliosis in Strasbourg within the Regional Health Agency of Alsace, that patients could get TicTox! This shows that the practice of phytotherapy was making headway, even among sceptics.

I also advise regular supplements of vitamin D, the anti-infective efficacy of which has been shown in tuberculosis and which has been shown to benefit autoimmune disease patients.

Various aspects of natural medicine would be worth professionalising and giving a code of practice; otherwise we run the risk of unscientific claims. For my part, I have always refused to participate in naturopathic meetings because of what I regard as unfounded 'certainties' and scandalous untruths about vaccines expressed at these, when all the evidence show these remain very safe and highly effective health products to which we owe our protection against many potentially serious diseases at all ages.

What happened to medical microbiology research?

First attempts at Lyme disease research

Sometime after my arrival in Garches in 1994 and faced with the influx of Lyme patients, I understood that there was a real medical and public health problem and that it was necessary to try to set up research projects. I saw more and more sick people come through and return to active life after years of suffering, fatigue and hardship. As two years before my arrival, the National Reference Centre (NRC) for Borreliosis had been transferred from Garches to the Pasteur Institute in Paris, and I myself, was deputy director of the National Reference Centre for Tuberculosis and Mycobacteria also located at the Pasteur Institute, I contacted Guy Baranton, the director of this Lyme centre.

In 1998, with his agreement, I organised a meeting of a few clinicians and researchers at the hospital in Garches. Baranton was a very good man, and a specialist in leptospires, but did not seem to have a particular passion for *Borreliae*. When, at the meeting, I explained that I was caring for desperate patients with chronic Lyme and that I was in contact with a patient association, I saw him turn white and he immediately told me that he did not want to 'play with this' and that chronic Lyme did not exist. He was sure since it was the Boston-based IDSA Lyme clique who had told him so. At least it had the virtue of being clear. We can see that, even in 2020, despite some agitation on my part, French research on the subject has remained at a standstill.

This is not for lack of submitting clinical and fundamental research projects for funding. Such funding is refused if the official dogma detailed in the IDSA text is not followed. Why fund research on an imaginary disease?

'Desperately seeking a researcher'

Microbes and communicable diseases have a mediaeval connotation in the imagination of researchers; they are diseases of the past. These professionals followed the analysis of the politicians and the great experts of the years 1970 to 1980. The 'real' diseases of the future were said to be immunological or genetic. Most research teams in large institutes have thus abandoned infection for other research considered 'more noble'. What a historic mistake! The only periods when some researchers show interest in infectious diseases is when epidemics or pandemics occur. We had the example of the H1-N1 influenza pandemic in 2009 and of the Covid-19 pandemic in 2020. Have them read Charles Nicolle again. Immunology is the study of the response to infections. Autoimmunity is probably the consequence of 'crypto-infections' not explained to date, provoking the immune system to attack the patient's own cells that are infected. Genetics plays a major role in susceptibility to infections and in the way the body controls them, but genetics does not explain all diseases. Even in diseases whose genetic cause is certain, such as familial Mediterranean fever (FMF) or myasthenia gravis, antibiotics can act on certain symptoms. I have often wondered if the well-known worsening of myasthenia with some antibiotics was not an exacerbation reaction.

If we listen to modern geriatricians, immuno-senescence (that is, the reduction of immune defences in the elderly) is paradoxically the consequence of hyper-stimulation of the immune system, which results in a significant increase in autoimmune phenomena. The 'crypto-infections' that accumulate in our organs with age must have something to do with it. During the Covid-19 pandemic, which was responsible for more severe cases in elderly people, there was no focus on the possible role of concomitant crypto-infections and what they might have contributed to susceptibility.

If we add to this 'antimicrobial fashion' a dose of polemic and an image of 'imaginary disease', how can we hope to find motivated researchers? The impossibility of obtaining funding for research and the censorship of Lyme publications have dramatic consequences for patients left to their fate. I have met some brilliant researchers who were enthusiastic about setting up research projects with me, but when they realised the problems, they preferred to turn towards research topics that were easier and, primarily, more rewarding, with the possibility of regular publications. Research directors reluctantly prefer to publish 'by the weight' dozens of articles whose scientific relevance is often mediocre and remain on the beaten track, rather than take risks in a real field of research that is far too random. I fully understand these colleagues and do not blame them for having abandoned me. Similarly, it is almost impossible for me to focus a young doctor at the beginning of their career on Lyme. That would be sending them straight into a brickwall and would definitely jeopardise their career. Fortunately, it was much easier for me to pursue research projects in other areas, such as hepatitis C and tuberculosis so my time has not been wasted.

Lyme and psychiatry

'Organic' and 'psychosomatic': the two muses of chronic disease

The mind clearly plays a part in, but is absolutely not the cause of Lyme disease, which is organic as we have seen. At the same time, 'real' psychiatric disorders do happen in Lyme patients due to inflammation of nerve tissue. I have seen some Lyme patients with acute psychosis, agitation, depression, obsessive-compulsive disorder and other conditions. Much more often, patients suffer from depression linked to a hellish daily existence, often filled with excruciating pain, exacerbated by isolation from and rejection by others, and with no visible way out. I have known patients who, as they could not see the light at the end of the tunnel, have killed themselves.

The mind can also have an effect on disease, as discussed in relation to Freud in Chapter 1. I have seen many sick people, who had evidently improved or even recovered, suddenly relapse within two weeks of a great stress, such as a death in the family, a car accident, a dismissal from their work or a separation. It is known that stress weakens the immune system.

As I was enthusiastic about the generally positive results of antibiotic treatments, I started talking to a few colleagues I knew well about this. Most of the time, after listening to me kindly for a few minutes, I would see their faces darken and they would look at me strangely as if I had lost my mind. I was facing a brickwall. One of my colleagues, whom I liked very much, laughed at me with one of her friends, saying that Garches had become the new Lourdes, with miracles being performed there, and that I was the new Bernadette Soubirous (who saw the Virgin Mary in the cave at Lourdes)! My patients, all regarded by others as having psychiatric problems', were being cured by a placebo effect or, better, a 'guru effect'. I don't know of many placebos – or 'gurus' that improve or cure 80% of people over extended periods of time. If such a remedy existed, I'd like to patent it!

Some doctors, in total denial, do a lot of harm to their patients with chronic Lyme. As I have said, they do not treat them for their pain, but label them psychosomatic hypochondriacs. Thus, many convince patients' families and their general practitioners that they are psychologically disturbed or faking their illness. I treated a woodcutter from the Vosges forest, who was badly handicapped and in pain, who had been ostracised from his village because he was considered a slacker, the worst insult for an Alsatian worker who loved his job. No-one had listened to him, including Social Security (our French health insurance), so he wanted to end his life. Shaking, he cried while telling me how he had been treated.

Among the deniers, the palm goes to a hospital doctor in the city of Mulhouse in eastern France, near the Swiss and German borders. I had heard a lot about this doctor from many patients for 15 years, because he had accused them of belonging to a cult. I did not know him, but I was not disappointed when I saw an interview with him in a report on Lyme disease. He said, with great assurance and a smirk, that the patients who complained of chronic Lyme were mostly fibromyalgic women who had been raped! Many patients talked regularly to me about this doctor because this derogatory statement shocked them a great deal.

I considered it a great honour when this colleague wrote to me for the first time in August 2015, a few days after the publication of my article in *La Presse Médicale* providing an objective critical review of publications on the treatment of chronic Lyme. He told me that, in his great experience with more than 1000 patients, he had cured all his Lyme patients in three weeks of treatment and that my article was a disgrace to French university medicine. Coming from him, I was very flattered to receive this attention!.

Another time, after I had spoken on a regional radio station, a doctor wrote to me, furious, telling me that I was reckless and that I had triggered an 'epidemic of hysterical false-Lyme'.

Whilst discussing my problem with the 'psychiatrification' of everything in modern medicine with a Belgian colleague, she said to me: 'Professor Perronne, do you know the difference between a psychiatrist and a locomotive?' As I confessed my ignorance she replied: 'When a locomotive goes off the rails, it stops!' I love Belgian humour.

Treating patients with chronic Lyme disease, even if it is complicated, has never been a problem for me personally. It was quite different with my colleagues in the department or elsewhere in the hospital. These patients were rejected and mocked by them, so much so that I hardly dared to have them hospitalised in my ward because I could hear residents and nurses say in the corridor: 'Ah, there's another one of Perronne's lunatics!' It was difficult to remain alone and misunderstood for years.

One day, I had to deal with a real psychiatric patient who arrived at my consultation in a state of acute psychosis. In her restless and disjointed speech, she nevertheless told me quite precisely about her journey to this point. She was married, had two small children, worked as a civil servant and had gone on vacation the previous summer to a 'bug- infested' rental home in the country. A few weeks later, she had developed meningitis.

She had been hospitalised in the Paris area where she had been diagnosed with viral meningitis and sent home. Her meningitis had gradually improved, but in the months that followed, she had developed episodes of fever, tremors, emotional instability and headaches, and then she had begun to feel pain in her joints, muscles and bones, as if they were being crushed. Then a permanent mental agitation developed, characteristic of a psychotic state.

As she had come alone for a consultation, this woman impressed me; she had obviously suffered a great deal yet was able, despite her apparent madness, to describe her medical problem with precision. I spoke about it to her doctor, and with her husband, and with the psychiatrist attached to the service so that he could calm her with antipsychotics which were essential given her state. I proposed admitting her to hospital to continue her on these drugs, but mostly to put her on antibiotic treatment. Of course, her Lyme antibody test came back negative, but this is so common – as we have seen – that it did not change my clinical reasoning. But at the sight of this result, the general practitioner preferred to ask for second opinions at two large departments of internal medicine in Paris, and renowned professors assured him that this woman was indeed mad, that chronic Lyme disease did not exist and that it was necessary to take away the custody of her children and to lock her up as quickly as possible, and for as long as possible, in a psychiatric unit so that she would not return and trouble her children anytime soon. The hospitalisation order, at the request of a third party, was signed without my knowledge. The patient, realising that she was going to be forcibly detained under mental health law, fled to her mother's home. She saw too she was about to lose the custody of her children. Crazy people are often very lucid!

When I heard about this, I was horrified. The police were after her, and the public prosecutor was on the case to have her sectioned. I fought through thick and thin to save this woman and her children, causing outrage in my own service. I felt my colleagues wanted to send me to mental hospital myself because I too was 'losing my mind and seeing Lyme everywhere'. One thing led to another, and I managed to have the patient hospitalised in my ward for antibiotic treatment. Of course, as expected, the treatment caused a violent exacerbation of her signs and symptoms at first, including her psychological state. It was hard for me to justify my 'obstinacy' with continuing treatment in the face of this 'manifest failure', but, after a few weeks, this patient finally recovered from her psychosis and the antipsychotics were gradually stopped. It took several months for the excruciating pain she was complaining of to disappear. This woman was able to keep her children and eventually found a job in a position of responsibility. Now, about 15 years on, she is still well and remembers this nightmare with emotion. When we see each other every two or three years, with hindsight we can laugh together about what happened.

Real or imagined pain?

I have many stories to tell about psychiatric patients. Many have told me that at the time they were sectioned they were suffering from excruciating pain that required morphine and that they spent their days and nights screaming they were in such agony. Psychiatrists, who did not believe they were in pain, were content with dulling them a little more with psychiatric drugs to get some peace. In less serious cases, I found that patients hospitalised in psychiatric departments for 'hysterical conversion' disorders (unexplained neurological deficits attributed to 'the mind') learned not to talk about their pain because, the pain being imaginary, verbalising it was a sign of regression! Some patients told me, after their recovery, that talking about their pain had very bad consequences and was a source of more severe abuse. When the psychiatrist asked them, 'How are you today?'

they were careful not to talk about their pain. The psychiatrist would then be happy, thinking that he had done a remarkable job on the patient's psyche, and consequently put less pressure on the patient.

Recently, as I mentioned in an earlier chapter (page 99), I managed to get a child out of a psychiatric ward in northern France – a 13-year-old boy who had been there for several months for 'hysterical conversion'. His parents had bought a house on the edge of the forest the previous year, and their son, top of his class and good at sport, regularly went into the forest to walk his dog. He had developed an erythema migrans that his mother had photographed and shown to their doctor, who had said it was nothing. A few months later, at the beginning of the school year, the boy had swollen lymph nodes and he could no longer run and then walk, and within a few months he had developed complete paraplegia with neurological damage to his bladder. His upper limbs were also beginning to be affected. The diagnosis of hysteria was confirmed in the largest paediatric hospital in Paris, the Necker Hospital. Once, the gendarmes had been sent to the parents' home to take the child by force, because they were accused of ill-treatment. Fortunately, the gendarmes had some insight and compassion and, noting the love and remarkable care of the parents, did not take him away. In the end the prosecutor dropped his initial decision to have him sectioned.

As the months went by, the child's condition got worse. Still hospitalised in the psychiatric ward, he was screaming with pain and had lost so much weight that he was all skin and bone. His mother thought of Lyme disease when she saw the remarkable film by Chantal Perrin (*Lyme Disease, a Silent Epidemic*), mentioned earlier in Chapter 7, which showed photos of erythema migrans. The psychiatrist did not want to hear about the mother's diagnosis. Rightly so, since, in his discourse, it was the parents who were the cause of their son's illness. Alerted by

Judith Albertat, then president of a patient association, I was able to hospitalise the boy at my hospital in Garches. By this stage he was a complete paraplegic and partially quadriplegic. After a few days of antibiotics, he was able to move his toes, his pain began to decrease and, after two months of antibiotics, he could walk again.

How many patients with 'crypto-infections' are there in psychiatric services in France, and even morearound the world? I am appalled by that thought. I have a small idea thanks to a patient who had stayed not far from Paris in a very chic and very expensive psychiatric clinic for the depressed of good family. She told me, as she knew Lyme symptoms well herself: 'They are all lymed in there', implying they all had neurological, joint, heart, skin, etc problems. The current situation is rather similar to what was observed before the antibiotic era, when a high proportion of patients in psychiatric hospitals had neuro-syphilis.

I have often wondered how some patients managed to resist committing suicide during this hellish psychiatric journey. A patient, whose doctor thought he was crazy and had convinced the patient's father to sign a request for psychiatric committal, told me, after his recovery, that he had repeatedly thought of suicide. He was locked in a cell on a bench in a psychiatric unit and, when the psychiatrist came in, he would curl up like a toad on a dissecting table. Unbearable pains were eating away at him day and night. He cried, asking for painkillers. The only answer he got from the psychiatrist was that these pains were all inside his head and that he had to improve his mental state. This patient had asked around and had thought about Lyme disease, but he had had negative antibody tests and was therefore unable to leave the 'psychiatry diagnostic box'. He was saved thanks to a Lyme antibody test performed by Mrs Schaller in Strasbourg (see page 102) who, outside official recommendations, practised using sensitive Western blots in cases of negative first-line Elisa tests. This practice is still banned as I have explained elsewhere in the book. As this patient's Lyme antibody test was found to be positive in the Schaller laboratory, he finally got a diagnosis.

Unfortunately, the doctors refused to give him antibiotics because the Schaller test was not officially recognised. As he did not have access to antibiotics, he started on treatment with TicTox, the herbal medicine that I have mentioned several times earlier – a mixture of essential oils from plants made by the pharmacist in Strasbourg, Bernard Christophe. Thanks to TicTox, this patient began to regain his health, and when I saw him in consultation a few months later, he had recovered half his strength. He was still very irritable on a psychological level. He had had such a traumatic time that, during his first consultation with me, he was still shaken with spasms and had crying fits. I was really upset when I saw this. Thanks to the antimicrobial treatment, he finally recovered. By letting him know that I admired him for the courage he had had, all alone, without any help from his family, to go through these terrible trials, he said to me: 'It was the illness that saved me. I didn't have the strength to get up and get a rope to hang myself'.' This supposedly crazy man has now recovered and is back working full time.

Most psychiatrists I have spoken to about these situations are in denial. They are not sick like Judith Mensch, the psychiatrist from Old Lyme who gave the alert in 1975. Many psychiatrists no longer practise physical medicine and do not even seek to link psychiatric disorders to a possible organic cause. Some only do psychoanalysis. I have, however, met psychiatrists of a different kind, especially in Germany. They had a solid background in physiology, internal medicine and neurology, and only treated mental symptoms in a holistic context. Fortunately, I do now meet French psychiatrists who have discovered chronic Lyme and who have totally changed their practices. One psychiatrist even recently admitted that she had started to do clinical examinations of her patients again, something she had not done for ages.

It is important, when treating a patient suffering from chronic Lyme disease for whom the signs are mainly subjective – i.e. based only on what the patient tells us – to try to find some objective signs to convince the general practitioner, the family and friends and the health insurance company, where relevant, of the physical reality of the disease. Jérôme Salomon, a doctor in my department, was one of my rare collaborators who believed in the existence of chronic Lyme, did as I did and accepted Lyme patients for consultations. With Jérôme and a resident, Marie-Odile Roche-Lanquetot, we published a study[19] showing that, when we looked hard, we could often find objective anomalies: decreased lymphocytes in the blood; abnormalities in the magnetic resonance imaging (MRI) scans of the brain or spinal cord; abnormalities in cognitive tests objectively measuring memory or concentration disorders; abnormalities in 'evoked potentials' that record the function of certain nerves; abnormalities, even discrete and non-specific, in the cerebrospinal fluid collected by lumbar puncture; etc. When the evidence is objective (visible to others and measurable) patients are less likely to be called crazy.

After the highly doubtful diagnoses of Münchhausen syndrome (that is, the simulation of disease to attract compassion/attention), which becomes a frequent 'easy' diagnosis, I have recently learned of terrible false accusations of 'Münchhausen syndrome by proxy'. This is a kind of transposition by which, instead of harming oneself to get attention as in Münchhausen's syndrome, one harms someone else – usually a child in one's family – to gain attention by deliberately making them ill. Recently, I discovered with dismay the crystallisation of terrible family tragedies in reaction to Lyme disease in children. As doctors could not explain the origin of symptoms, family members would sometimes come up with diabolical theories. For example, a father accused his ex-wife of poisoning their daughter; in another case, a grandmother suspected her daughter of poisoning her own children. These cases have gone far, with 'testimonies' from doctors and social workers, and harassment from judges. I had to intervene several times to stop the withdrawal of parental custody before I could successfully treat children with antibiotics.

We need to revisit dogmas

Neither God Nor Genes, *a key book for understanding medicine*

Pierre Sonigo is a friend who, as a young researcher, contributed to the sequencing of the HIV virus in Luc Montagnier's laboratory at the Institut Pasteur. I first came across him in the late 1990s at a scientific meeting on AIDS. Pierre gave a scientific presentation that was both simple and dazzlingly clear, which is the privilege of the great. It was the first time I had heard about HIV disease with such clarity. Sometime later, I discovered the book he had written with Jean-Jacques Kupiec entitled *Ni Dieu ni Gène (Neither God Nor Genes).* This book, along with Charles Nicolle's *Le Destin des Maladies Infectieuses (The Destiny of Infectious Diseases),* mentioned earlier (see page 321), and Sagan and Margulis' *Microcosmos,* are the books that have changed my vision of medicine and infectious diseases the most. The language of Sonigo's book is so simple and full of imagery that one thinks one is reading 'immunology for children'.

In fact, this work based on very advanced scientific knowledge explains, among other things, how the immune cells of 'Monsieur Dupont' (the French equivalent of the proverbial 'Mr Smith') don't care about Monsieur Dupont who they are not acquainted with. Like all cells on the planet, their sole purpose is to feed, survive and reproduce. If a white blood cell belonging to Mr Dupont swallows a bacterium, it is not to defend him from a serious infection; it is only to feed itself. Indeed, microbial antigens (the specific chemical structures on the surface of the microbe) are excellent snacks for immune cells. So called 'autoimmunity' is the consequence of tissue infection. If Mr Dupont's elbow joint becomes painful, hot, red and swollen (*dolor, calor, rubor, tumor* in Latin, the cardinal signs of inflammation), it is because immune cells, including some white blood cells, have converged there. They have come in numbers because there is food. And what do these cells eat? Microbial antigens!

The discipline of immunology was born at the time of the bitter rivalry between France and Germany at the end of the nineteenth century, and military comparisons were used to explain defences against infections, as if the immune cells were small soldiers gathered in army corps, under the orders of their owner, Monsieur Dupont, to drive out invaders. This vision was revived by the Franco-German rivalry between the schools of Louis Pasteur and Robert Koch. This simplistic warlike image of immunity has been taken up by many AIDS specialists. Jacques Leibowitch, in his book *Pour en Finir avec le Sida (How to End AIDS)*, questioned this pseudo-consensus and clearly showed that it is the body's inflammatory responses and not the HIV virus itself that create lesions in the body's tissues leading to AIDS symptoms. Leibowitch evokes competition for 'food' between human cells and microbes. It was this highly innovative approach that enabled him to develop the HIV treatment reduction strategy, ICCARRE, that I will expand on below, and that was recently confirmed in a formal therapeutic trial I coordinated at the National AIDS Research Agency (ANRS), the 4D trial (short for 'four days' a week' of treatment).

Chapter 9

Crypto-infections

Many diseases could be triggered by 'crypto-infections'

The concept of 'crypto-infections' seems to apply to more and more medical situations. We have seen constant new discoveries that show the link between this or that microbe and this or that disease. Taking the lead from Charles Nicolle (see page 134), some Pasteur supporters have taken up the idea that chronic diseases of unexplained origin could be linked to 'silent infections'. Among them are Professor Paul Giroud of the Pasteur Institute, who was Charles Nicolle's assistant, and Professor Jean-Baptiste Jadin of the Prince Leopold Institute of Antwerp in Belgium, who built up enormous experience as a field researcher in the former Belgian colonies of Congo-Kinshasa and Rwanda. In the 1980s they described associations of certain diseases with protozoans (single-cell parasites), viruses and bacteria. They mentioned the possible role of intracellular bacteria, especially *Rickettsiae* and *Rickettsia*-like bacteria, as well as *Chlamydiae.*

I remember very well, during my senior registrar period in the old Claude-Bernard Hospital (see page 38), that a woman with an unexplained chronic syndrome was admitted to hospital. She had had a *Rickettsia* antibody test in Belgium developed by Jadin and Giroud, which had been positive. With this result, she had been prescribed tetracycline which had considerably improved her condition. However, as these Belgian tests were not officially recognised in France, her doctor had refused to extend the treatment. The professor of infectious diseases who oversaw the clinic at the time explained to me that such patients were fantasist hypochondriacs who were going to Belgium to seek fraudulent tests in order to be prescribed antibiotics unjustifiably. The situation was similar to cases at that time of chronic brucellosis (called brucellian fatigue), where the patients were viewed as lazy freeloaders on health insurance.

These old stories are reminiscent of the current situation. Jean-Baptiste Jadin's daughter, Cécile Jadin, is a doctor herself and spent her entire childhood in Africa working with her father. She has told me that she would often go along with him to the laboratory. The family house was filled with experimental animals. Cécile moved to South Africa in 1981 as a surgeon. In 1987, she took care of one of her friends with chronic fatigue syndrome who had lost the ability to walk. Since then, she had devoted herself to the management of many chronic diseases with antimicrobial medicines. When I spoke with her, I was impressed by her experience. She was doing such a fantastic job that it got her... attacked by the South African Medical Association Council! She has rescued people with serious illnesses who were failing to recover with 'official' treatments. She still continues to treat very diverse symptomatologies. I met her in 2016 in Belgium and she amazed me by letting me listen to the voice of one of her patients on her smartphone, who had been stuttering for several years, making his diction very difficult, even incomprehensible at times. She then made me listen to the voice of the same man after a few weeks of antibiotics. He spoke very normally!

It is highly likely that, in chronic diseases, all types of microbes can be involved: viruses, bacteria, parasites, fungi. It's a fascinating world.

Chapter 9

My fascination with mycobacteria, responsible for persistent infections

When I started out in research my interest focused on a major scourge, tuberculosis, caused by Koch's bacillus *(Mycobacterium tuberculosis*) and on related bacteria and atypical mycobacteria which contributed to the death of one out of two patients when AIDS was advanced.

During my years at the Claude-Bernard Hospital, and then in Bichat, tuberculosis was ravaging patients infected with HIV. In addition, many patients who died of advanced AIDS had infections with bacteria similar to the tuberculosis bacillus in all their organs; these were much less virulent, atypical mycobacteria, mainly *Mycobacterium avium.* These bacteria are widespread in the environment, especially in water , and in some animals, and do not usually cause disease in healthy humans. On the other hand, patients with AIDS, who no longer had immune defences, very often had severe forms of infection that were often fatal. Conventional anti-tuberculosis treatments did not work or did not work very well. Working in an INSERM laboratory, as I have described, in the former Claude-Bernard Hospital to test new antibiotics on these bacteria, I then worked with some colleagues to develop new effective treatments against these mycobacteria. These new treatments have enabled us to treat many AIDS patients.

From mycobacteria to granulomatous diseases: sarcoidosis and Crohn's disease

While I was carefully studying all the new and old scientific publications on mycobacteria, I realised that some autoimmune diseases – called granulomatous diseases – looked very much like some forms of tuberculosis or atypical mycobacterial infections. Among these diseases, the best known are sarcoidosis (an inflammatory lung disease) and Crohn's disease (an inflammatory bowel disease).

I discovered that, in the tissues of patients suffering from sarcoidosis, certain mycobacteria, most often not tuberculous, could be isolated. These bacteria seemed to be structured without any cell wall (L forms). Bacteria without a cell wall do not take up the usual colourings ('stains') used for identification and are therefore not visible under the microscope. I was struck by seeing that two people managed to contract sarcoidosis at the same time after a bath in a jacuzzi, and that an atypical mycobacterium was isolated in the lung of one of these two patients thanks to bronchial fibroscopy. A study showed a close correlation between sarcoidosis and the presence of antimycobacterial antibodies. A link was also shown with *Chlamydia* infections. In support of a possible infective cause of the disease, one could note that nursing personnel are affected preferentially. It is troubling to note also that sarcoidosis has not shown an increase in the French West Indies (Antilles), but that it has increased among people from the Antilles who have lived in mainland France. That suggests environmental factors.

With regard to Crohn's disease, I had read an old study that showed that in an area where cattle herds were heavily affected by a condition called Johne's disease, there were outbreaks of Crohn's disease among the population from villages living downstream from the fields occupied by these herds. Johne's disease is characterised by severe diarrhoea in cattle and is due to the atypical mycobacterium, *Mycobacterium avium subspecies para-tuberculosis*. Crohn's disease is mainly a digestive disease characterised by diarrhoea. This mycobacterium has been isolated numerous times from the colon walls of patients affected by Crohn's. High milk consumption is correlated with the frequency of the condition, but the bacterium may also be present in water. Cases of transmission of Crohn's disease have been reported in couples. The culture of *Mycobacterium avium subspecies paratuberculosis* is very long and requires liquid culture media that must be kept for at least four to six months to have a chance of isolating the bacterium. This is why it is never isolated in current practice. The bacterium can also be isolated by polymerase chain reaction (PCR).

For Crohn's disease, the criteria of Henle-Koch's postulate (or 'Koch's postulate': 'one microbe, one disease') are met with the attribution of Crohn's to this mycobacterium, as shown by Greenstein in the journal *Lancet Infectious Diseases* in 2003.[103] However, this has not in the least shaken the gastroenterologists who continue to speak of it as an 'autoimmune' disease. It is true that two very powerful lobbies, those of the milk and the pharmaceutical industries, do not want things to change. Indeed, the new immunosuppressive treatments for Crohn's disease and sarcoidosis cost the health service a fortune and are prescribed for life. To top it all off, some patients develop both sarcoidosis and Crohn's disease.

Some granulomatous diseases could be treated and even cured with antimicrobials

At that time, I offered an antimycobacterial antibiotic treatment to a patient suffering from very severe sarcoidosis whose spleen had become monstrous. (The spleen is part of the immune system. She had been advised that she had to have her spleen removed and go on heavy immunosuppressive treatment. She was delighted with my proposal because she had nothing to lose. One month after starting antibiotic treatment, her health had improved considerably, and her spleen volume had decreased significantly. Strengthened by this success, I treated and cured several patients.

I had spoken about these therapeutic successes to Professor Jacques Grosset, an eminent specialist in tuberculosis and mycobacteria with whom I collaborated for my work on

Mycobacterium avium. He had dissuaded me at the time from publishing these cases of sarcoidosis by telling me that nobody would believe me and that the specialists in the disease would speak of 'spontaneous remission'. (On this point, I saw later that he was entirely right.)

'Mycosarc': the antibiotic treatment trial for sarcoidosis

I later developed an official protocol, called 'Mycosarc' (for mycobacteria and sarcoidosis), that the Pasteur Institute promoted in 1996. The aim was to evaluate the efficacy of an antibiotic by comparing it with a placebo in volunteer patients. I had presented my patients' files to the greatest specialists in sarcoidosis who listened to me and promised that they would participate in this research with me. I even presented on the small series of patients I had treated at the annual conference of the French National Society of Internal Medicine. In particular, I showed the scans of the patient who had had a monstrous spleen before it returned to almost normal after a few months of antimicrobial treatment. I saw some smirks in the front rows of the audience. Then radio silence! These investigating colleagues never included a single patient in the protocol. So, the study never came to a successful conclusion, and later some people said that this treatment strategy did not work. I was annoyed but could not do anything because at the time the internet was not yet very developed, and I had no personal patients with sarcoidosis I could recruit. As with all chronic diseases, patients enter organised care channels from which they can rarely escape.

The same scenario was repeated with Crohn's disease. With Professor Patrick Berche, a famous microbiologist, who was later Dean of the Necker Faculty of Medicine and who eventually headed the Pasteur Institute in Lille, we set up a treatment protocol for Crohn's disease. Collaborating gastroenterologists imposed unrealistic microbiological evaluation criteria and the study had to be stopped quickly.

I didn't blame all those colleagues – respiratory physicians and gastroenterologists, all excellent doctors otherwise with whom I had very friendly relationships. They were not ready to challenge entrenched dogma: a disease is infectious, in which case the microbe is easily found, or it is not. So, I abandoned that research, but occasionally, as a service, I continued to treat patients with sarcoidosis with antimicrobials, almost all of whom got better.

My experience with Crohn's disease is limited to a small number of patients. The first patient I treated with antimicrobials was a general practitioner who had heard of my anti-infection approach. For many years he had suffered from severe Crohn's with terrible abdominal pain, very frequent diarrhoea during the day in addition to severe fatigue and joint problems. He took a large dose of a cortisone derivative orally every day and had to perform a daily colon enema with corticosteroids. He was so ill despite this heavy treatment that his gastroenterologist was about to introduce a new immunosuppressive drug.

Initially, I was not very keen to treat him because, unlike sarcoidosis, I had never treated Crohn's disease. He begged me to help him and, as he was a doctor himself, I was reassured I could go through this experience with him. Within a few weeks, his condition had changed, and after a few months, he gradually and permanently stopped his enemas and steroids. He had completely recovered. His treatment combined clarithromycin, rifabutin and ethambutol, ethambutol being replaced by hydroxychloroquine after three months. When he saw his gastroenterologist, a great Parisian Crohn's professor, again to tell him about the result of my treatment, I was surprised to receive a letter from this professor telling me that the patient had benefited from a 'spontaneous remission'. When I showed this letter to my patient, we both laughed. Those who believe in 'spontaneous generation' (see page 18) are also fans of 'spontaneous remissions'!

I then treated a small number of other patients. One patient, after an initial dramatic improvement, stopped their treatment. Another stopped his treatment after a few days due to a significant increase in transaminases – liver enzymes. He did not want to try the experiment again with alternative drugs. The others, who suffered from severe forms treated by immunosuppressants, were cured and some have been able to go several years without treatment.

As I researched into Crohn's disease, I discovered more censorship and blindness in the field of scientific thought and publication. This is illustrated, among many other things, by the fate of a paper by Gerald Gui, in 1997, which is a superb English study conducted in 52 patients suffering from Crohn's disease. This study showed the efficacy in all patients of the combination of two antibiotics active on mycobacteria: clarithromycin (or azithromycin) and rifabutin. As this study had not been carried out by randomly giving a placebo to some patients (a method called 'randomised double blind'), it was not even read by gastroenterologists. A case of double-blind blindness! Yet the majority of patients in this study had not responded to conventional Crohn's treatments at the beginning of the trial and their follow-up lasted two years. These must of course be more 'spontaneous remissions'! One or two is possible, I would agree, but more than 50 at once is a higher rate than the frequency of miracles observed at Lourdes.

This study was not included in a meta-analysis (overall analysis of all published articles on the subject) by Feller in 2010 because it was not randomised. The meta-analysis only cited studies that had used antibiotics (metronidazole, fluoroquinolones, etc) that could improve patients' condition but not cure them. Meanwhile, millions of Crohn's disease patients (and the disease is said to be on the rise) receive life-long immunosuppressive treatments at exorbitant cost and experience the joys of digestive surgery.

I was very surprised recently when a patient with Crohn's disease came to see me for antibiotic treatment. I told him about my experience and when I told him that I had cured some patients, he got scared because it was totally unimaginable for him. He left quickly and I never saw him again. He must have thought I was crazy. It is very difficult for a patient to come out of institutional conditioning.

Unexpected insights into autism, schizophrenia and Alzheimer's disease

Behind the scenes of autism

At the presentation of the Nobel Prize in Physiology or Medicine to Luc Montagnier, discoverer of the HIV virus, I met a group of general practitioners, the Chronimed group, whose members had built up an excellent knowledge of the management of chronic Lyme, but also of other chronic diseases, notably certain psychiatric conditions. Thus, Philippe Bottero is a general practitioner from Nyons in the Drôme department of France who at the beginning of his career had met Professor Jean-Baptiste Jadin, Belgian researcher at the Prince-Léopold Institute in Antwerp, and Colonel Paul Le Gac of the French colonial troops. From them, Philippe Bottero learned the possible link between chronic silent infections and chronic diseases. He became aware of work published by Loo and Menier in 1960 in the *Annales de Médecine Physiologique* on the possible link between intracellular bacteria and neuropsychiatric diseases.

Philippe Bottero is a pioneer for me because he was the first, all alone in his general practice, to improve and even cure people suffering from schizophrenia, manic-depressive psychosis, obsessive-compulsive disorders and autism by prolonged antibiotic therapies. In 2006, he met Dr Philippe Raymond, a general practitioner who was treating an impressive succession of autistic children. Since then, these two doctors have had followers and we know that with the involvement of a whole group of motivated general practitioners and psychiatrists, who trained among themselves, hundreds of French autistic children have improved or lost all their autistic symptoms thanks to their antimicrobial treatments. The treatment seems to work much better when the condition is recent. The effectiveness of antibiotics in intermittent cures is enhanced by short courses of antiparasitic and antifungal agents, as well as with a low-gluten diet. These autism specialists found that children often had digestive problems before they developed signs of autism. This is disturbing when we know that we can find in the faeces of people with autism, bacteria such as *Sutarella sp.* and *Ruminococcus sp* that are mostly absent from the digestive tracts of healthy people.

These doctors invited me to one of their meetings and I was impressed by the autistic children's records that they showed me. Since they could not convince hospital doctors, especially child psychiatrists, they started filming the behaviour of autistic children before and after treatment, and it is wonderful to see a child who was screaming, refusing any contact with friends and family, or banging his head against the walls, change his behaviour completely after a few weeks of an antibiotic, azithromycin. The same child began to follow with his eyes, to be much calmer and to play with an educator, starting to smile for the first time.

These accounts are deeply moving. Philippe Raymond asked me to help him publish his experience and, especially, to set up an official clinical study that would validate his work by comparing an antibiotic with a placebo. So, I went with him in 2011 to meet Dr Nadia Chabane, a child psychiatrist at the Robert-Debré University Hospital in Paris. Nadia Chabane was one of the hospital doctors in France who saw great numbers of autistic children in consultation. Many, if not almost all, child psychiatrists thought Philippe Raymond and his colleagues were charlatans. Nadia Chabane on the other hand seemed convinced by his work because she had reviewed several of the children who had received antibiotics. After several recoveries, it seemed difficult to continue to say that it was an exceptional spontaneous remission or that it was the mother who had improved her contact with her child. It must be said that psychotherapy, which continues to be covered by France's Social Security health payments, has never cured a single case of autism.

Philippe Raymond invited me to accompany him and Luc Montagnier to a meeting with advisors of Xavier Bertrand, then Minister of Social Affairs. I could not attend the meeting, but the result was very positive. The ministry was going to ask for research funds to be earmarked for a clinical study, and Xavier Bertrand's advisers asked Professor Nicholas Moore, director of the pharmacology department at Bordeaux University Hospital, to coordinate the study. Several committed university hospital child psychiatrists agreed to participate. In 2012, I helped Philippe Raymond and Nicholas Moore write the first draft of a project called 'Autibiotics' for autism and antibiotics. The efficacy of an antibiotic would be evaluated for a few months against a placebo, then, if the efficacy of the treatment was confirmed, the children receiving the placebo would receive the antibiotic in a second phase.

By chance, the presidential elections then arrived, and the Minister for Health changed. The cabinet of the new Minister, Marisol Touraine, as well as that of the Secretary of State for Higher Education and Research, Geneviève Fioraso, did not believe in the relevance of the project unlike their predecessors, and no funding was released. During the following years, the blockage persisted not only on autism, but more generally on Lyme disease and associated diseases. For autism, it is a particular pity because, even if the treatment does not work in all children, its effectiveness could be demonstrated quite quickly with a few dozen patients.

In fact, this project came at a time when France's High Authority for Health (HAS) was publishing its report on psychoanalysis in autism. The report was leaked in the newspaper *Libération* in February 2012, angering French psychoanalysts who had been lobbying hard. The report indeed said that psychoanalysis was useless in autism and that it was necessary to stop recommending it and therefore covering payments for it. In the face of the outcry from the psychoanalists and under pressure, the final version of the HAS report was, to general surprise, much more conciliatory. The psychoanalysts had reason to rejoice at the burial of the Autibiotic project. The 100% coverage of psychoanalysis for autism by Social Security was maintained despite the lack of therapeutic results for more than a century!

New perspectives in schizophrenia

As with autism, many doctors around the world have observed improvement in schizophrenic patients after antibiotic treatments. Right now, official psychiatry does not want to hear about it. It seems chronic diseases that are not cured represent a good income situation for many. However, randomised double-blind placebo-controlled studies (the 'gold standard' for such research as mentioned earlier) have been published demonstrating the, at least partial and transient, efficacy of antibiotics. So, even studies conducted according to the best modern methodological standards are ignored when they show a result that disturbs established prejudices. Medical ethics should require the continuation of this promising research.

Troubling Alzheimer's research results confirmed

Thanks to my meeting with Judith Miklossy, a Swiss researcher working in Valais, I was able to shed light on another aspect of

Lyme disease, in particular – its incestuous links with tertiary (late stage) syphilis and Alzheimer's disease. I discovered that at the very beginning of the Lyme saga, an American researcher, Alan MacDonald (whom I met at the Oslo conference – see page 127), had found that the *Borrelia burgdorferi* bacterium could escape antibiotics by taking a different form from the characteristic spiral; this was a round form, initially named a 'cystic form', but it was found not really to be a cyst, clearly visible under a microscope. This discovery was not at all in line with the IDSA verses and Alan MacDonald was discredited. This is strange because the Brorson brothers in Norway, as well as Professor Laane, still in Norway, have published on these round forms. Judith Miklossy, taking up MacDonald's work, has also described them. For Steere, Wormser et al, the leaders of the the IDSA expert group, all these researchers were impostors who were imagining things and the images they had all observed under the microscope were not forms of *Borrelia* but artefacts – that is, specks of dirt – because these people did not know how to conduct their research properly. What scientific impudence!

Thanks to Alan MacDonald's and Judith Miklossy's publications, I discovered that, when one puts side by side under the microscope, brain sections from patients who have died from three different diseases, the microscopic images are identical. These three diseases are neuro-syphilis, neuro-Lyme and Alzheimer's disease.

Alois Alzheimer was a German neurologist, who was also a psychiatrist and anatomopathologist. In 1901 he observed the first case of the disease that now bears his name. It was his laboratory boss, Emil Kraepelin, who suggested the name Alzheimer's disease. Kraepelin wanted to prove the superiority of his anatomical school over psychoanalytic theories and wanted to pull the rug out from under Sigmund Freud to show that certain mental disorders could have an organic origin and that not everything was psychosomatic. Kraepelin was a visionary.

At the time, many people in Europe were suffering from syphilis and there were many cases of tertiary syphilis. The form reaching the brain was called 'general paresis' or paralysis. It was not really paresis or a paralysis in most cases, but a form of dementia that was sometimes early. We know that General Gamelin, commander in chief of the French armed forces before the beginning of the Second World War and who shared responsibility for the rout of 1940, was affected by it. Alzheimer himself, noting the similarities in silver colouration between cerebral neuro-syphilis and the disease that bears his name, would also have noted the similarity of the clinical signs of dementia between the two diseases. After the discovery of *Treponema pallidum*, the infective agent causing syphilis, he would have said that 'his' disease, Alzheimer's, was probably also an infectious disease whose microbe could not yet be detected. This hypothesis was given new life in 1907 by Fischer who tried in vain to highlight a bacterium.

Alois Alzheimer quoted Fischer's work in 1911, and Judith Miklossy cites this historical data in a 2015 publication.[159] It is curious that the many researchers around the world, who receive a lot of money to do research about the cause of Alzheimer's disease, do not go back and read Fischer and Alzheimer again. This is 'collective Alzheimer's' (or is it epidemic?). The postulation of infectious causes for diseases always disturbs the relevant medical specialists. Alan MacDonald first, then Judith Miklossy, found the same similarities between the two conditions but in addition they found exactly the same appearance in a third condition, in the brains of people who died of late Lyme disease with brain damage and dementia. In a huge study involving hundreds of brains, Judith was able to formally demonstrate that Alzheimer's disease was a neuro-spirochetosis (a neurological disease caused by a spirochete infection), meaning that more than 90% of people who die of Alzheimer's disease have brains stuffed with little spring-like bacteria such as *Treponema* and/or

Borrelia. When she analysed 'control brains' from people who had died of another disease, she did not find the spirochetes. These results meet the famous criteria of Henle-Koch's postulate mentioned above and later modified by Hill, which allows us to affirm that spirochetes are the cause of Alzheimer's disease.

What spirochetes are responsible for this condition? In a quarter of cases it is *Borrelia burgdorferi* (bizarre for a supposedly rare infection) and in three quarters of cases, non-syphilitic *Treponemae* originating from dental plaque. If the study had been made in the nineteenth century or early twentieth century, one would surely have found in addition many *Treponema pallidum* organisms, the causative agent of syphilis. While these works have been published, and many experiments have been reproduced in different laboratories, it is curious, to say the least, to note the deafening silence around this major discovery, both on the part of the 'official specialists' on Lyme and on the part of microbiologists and neurologists.

Some epidemiologists and dentists have investigated the issue because there is now a proven link between very damaged gums, spoiled teeth and Alzheimer's disease. Yet these non-syphilitic *Treponemae,* known as saprophytes (resident organisms not known to cause disease), live in large quantities in dental plaque. At a conference on Lyme disease in Germany, I heard an exciting talk by an English stomatologist and maxillofacial surgeon, Professor St John Crean, Dean of the School of Medicine and Dentistry at the University of Central Lancashire, who was studying a possible link between Alzheimer's and dental plaque bacteria. He had found derivatives of *Porphyromonas gingivalis,* a plaque bacterium, in the brains of people who had died of Alzheimer's disease.

I am very surprised, when we see the hundreds of millions of pounds injected into Alzheimer's research around the world that no one talks about this, not even for a second, even though this work indicates that Alzheimer's disease is an infectious disease.

As for the cases of Alzheimer's disease due to Lyme infection, these must amount to a great many given it is currently predicted that 80% of people in Europe will develop Alzheimer's disease. If even only a quarter of this 80% is due to *Borrelia*, we are no longer looking at the rare disease registry.

I remember that, when I was a neurology student in the service of Professor Jean Cambier at Beaujon Hospital in 1976, Alzheimer's disease was still described as an uncommon disease. Some neurologists talked about 'microtubule diseases' because pathologists observed a micro-fibrillary degeneration of the brain. The neuro-fibrils observed inside nerve cells result from the aggregation of microtubules. When I learned in 2000, by reading Sagan and Margulis' book *Microcosmos*, that our cells are built around the microtubules of spirochetes, I immediately made the connection.

Would it be conceivable that, when a spirochete like *Treponema pallidum*, agent of syphilis, or a *Borrelia*, agent of Lyme disease, or a non-syphilitic *Treponema* in dental plaque, entered the cells of our brain, it created a mess with its atypical microtubules among the microtubules of our cells? Scientific publications on Alzheimer's are of course totally ignored by the Lyme clique of IDSA. Rightly so, since Lyme is an imaginary disease!

Unfortunately for deniers, Alan MacDonald's and Judith Miklossy's results have more recently been confirmed by another team based in Philadelphia, whose study was published in 2016 and showed the respective roles of spirochetes, biofilms and the immune reaction in the brains of Alzheimer's disease patients.[24]

In 2009, a woman, Fabienne Piel, shared her medical journey in a French context. A renowned dog breeder, she began suffering from memory problems at the age of 37. After initial hypotheses suggesting overwork or depression, a diagnosis came after a few years: Alzheimer's disease. She recounted her ordeal in her book *J'ai Peur d'Oublier* (*I Fear Forgetting*) and created an organisation called *La Vie Sans Oubli* (*Life Without Forgetting*). Years later, then very ill, she heard about Dr Philippe Bottero, the pioneering general practitioner from Nyons who, in this case again, would demonstrate his talent. He treated Fabienne with antibiotics and she was cured from her 'Alzheimer's disease' in a few months. This fantastic story was reported in June 2016 in *Paris Match* magazine. The fact that the disease occurred so early in life could explain why the neurons were preserved, allowing recovery.

While this miracle was happening, the local council of the Order of Physicians found Philippe Bottero guilty of charlatanism. He, who was so appreciated by his patients, was deeply affected by this decision. A conviction for a doctor who is dangerous or abuses his patients, can be understood, especially when there is a complaint from them. In the Lyme affair, there had never been a complaint from patients, but on the contrary an accumulation of messages of support and thanks. In the face of the evidence clearly demonstrating the bacterial cause of certain cases of Alzheimer's disease, confirmed by different research teams, not acknowledging these objective facts was – and remains – completely incomprehensible to a scientific mind. As I have said, it is likely that the treatment was effective in Fabienne because she was young. Antibiotics are unlikely to have much effect in elderly people with advanced Alzheimer's disease, who have often lost almost half of their brain mass by the time of diagnosis. Destroyed nerve cells do not grow back. Prevention should be done upstream.

The key message for prevention is to avoid tick bites. In gardens, parks, grassy areas and forests, repellents can be used, either chemical products sold in pharmacies, or natural biological repellents. If bitten, a tick-remover should be slipped under the tick's head, without queezing its body, and an antiseptic must be applied on the bite site, after removal of the tick. Look for the appearance of a 'bull's eye' rash – if this appears, the physician must prescribe an appropriate antibiotic treatment for at least two weeks.

Could other 'non-infectious' chronic conditions be caused by crypto-infections?

As a result of accumulating experience of prolonged antimicrobial treatments in many and varied clinical cases, I realised that an incredible number of manifestations, a priori not at all known for their infectious origin, could respond to antibiotic or antiparasitic treatment. For example, I have seen thyroid nodules regress or disappear. In a few patients whose radiologists had identified so-called 'idiopathic' or 'functional' cysts of the liver, spleen or kidney, these had disappeared. As noted above, the medical term 'idiopathic' is used for a disease whose cause is unknown. Official medicine also attributes certain diseases to cold. In particular, the many cases of facial paralysis that appear from nowhere without any identifiable cause. These may well be cases of Lyme disease with negative antibody tests, or even the result of other co-infections. However, we still call these facial paralyses (Bell's palsy) *a frigore* Latin for a 'cold snap'! The same was said of 'influenza', or 'flu', before the discovery of influenza viruses. This term comes from the popular Italian name *influenza di freddo,* which means 'under the influence of the cold'.

The list of disorders that can respond to antimicrobial medicines is impressive. Asthma regresses or disappears in some patients. In this field, Professor Dominique Gendrel, a leading paediatrician at Saint-Vincent-de-Paul Hospital, showed in a publication that children suffering from chronic asthma were long-term hosts of intracellular bacteria, *Chlamydia* and *Mycoplasma,* in their bronchi.[37]

Allergies, recurrent herpes, chronic or recurrent ENT infections, psoriasis, Raynaud's syndrome, carpal tunnel syndrome, chronic tendonitis, sciatica or cervico-brachial neuralgia, osteoarthritis, migraines, various mood disorders, sleep disorders, visual disorders (many of which include uveitis, retinitis, optic nerve neuritis, etc), digestive disorders, tachycardia onsets, including known cases of Bouveret tachycardia, recurrent pericarditis, recurrent canker sores, Hashimoto's thyroiditis, rebellious chronic itching, endometriosis, sclero-atrophic lichen, chronic pancreatitis, restless leg syndrome, narcolepsy and hepatic steatosis have decreased or disappeared (often after initial worsening of symptoms) with antimicrobial therapy. I have seen clear improvements in some diseases, such as ankylosing spondylitis, familial Mediterranean fever (FMF) and Parkinson's disease. I remember a woman whose blood lipids (cholesterol and especially triglycerides) increased enormously in the first month of treatment before returning to the normal range. A diabetic insulin-dependent man saw his diabetes unbalanced for a week or two and then his insulin needs were cut in half.

I was amazed to see these incredible results that I could not have expected. When I sometimes tried to talk to a few colleagues about these findings, they all looked at me in a bewildered way as if it was so stupid that it was not even worth talking about. So, I bit my tongue! I have seen recovery from very real autoimmune diseases: lupus, rheumatoid arthritis, Still's disease, multiple sclerosis, transverse myelitis, amyotrophic lateral sclerosis, histiocytosis, idiopathic lymphocytopenia, monoclonal gammapathy, TRAPS (TNF-receptor associated periodic syndrome, a relapsing fever linked to a genetic anomaly), Behçet's disease, Horton's disease. Some patients sadly relapsed partially a few years later.

I would not want to give false hope to people suffering from any of these diseases because antimicrobials can affect many diseases but most often they are not enough to recover from them. It is out of the question to put everyone on antibiotics for everything and anything because this massive and abusive use would have serious consequences for bacterial resistance. However, these observations show that, if we had at our disposal effective tests enabling us to predict who will improve with which drug and how, we could target prescriptions. We also know that non-antibiotic drugs can have an effect and, as described in the previous chapter, therapies using natural products such as phytotherapy could be used for prevention.

I have tried to publish on some of these cases, in particular a case of TRAPS. A man had had an ongoing series of fevers of 39°C each lasting for several days, every month for years and had consulted doctors throughout Paris. His life had become a living hell. In the light of the fever's relapsing profile, I treated him with antibiotics and hydroxychloroquine, and he recovered permanently in four months. The TRAPS mutation was unknown at the time. I had requested a genetic search for familial Mediterranean fever, which was negative. Years later, I received a letter from the genetics laboratory informing me that they had re-analysed samples kept in the freezer and that this patient had the TRAPS mutation, only discovered since its collection. As I had not seen this man for years, I checked up on him and informed him of the retrospective diagnosis. He was still in great shape and had never had a fever again. This account of TRAPS was 'trapped' by the medical journals telling me that it was nonsense and that it was not based on known evidence or recommendations. And for a very good reason. Finally, in 2020, I succeeded in publishing this case.[5]

A striking family story: the same ticks cause three different chronic diseases

A young woman who had a severe form of Behçet's disease with recurrent meningitis and encephalitis, regular fevers of 40°C, and joint, eye and digestive problems associated with mouth and genital sores, was 23 years old and had fallen ill as a child at the age of nine, after being bitten by ticks during her summer holidays. She had presented with a huge erythema (bull's eye rash). A month later, she had been hospitalised in paediatric intensive care in Garches for meningo-encephalitis for which no cause could be found at the time and that had been treated as possible tuberculous meningitis. The anti-tuberculosis treatment contained the drug rifampicin, active against *Borrelia*, and this is probably what cured her at the time.

I later learned that two of her sisters also had a chronic disease: one had 'seronegative' rheumatoid arthritis (i.e. with no rheumatoid factor, the official marker of the disease), and the other had chronic fatigue syndrome with fibromyalgia. Her mother then told me that the three sisters had all become ill at the same time in childhood and that ticks had been removed two weeks before the onset of their diseases. While the first sister was hospitalised in intensive care for her meningo-encephalitis, another of the sisters had also been hospitalised in Garches, but in another department, the paediatric orthopaedic surgery department, for acute tibial osteomyelitis. The surgeon had operated on her and the bone analysis had found some inflammation but not the usual lesions of osteomyelitis, while bacteria could not be isolated in culture. She had recovered at the time with an antibiotic. I was very moved to read in the archives of Garches Hospital the two medical files from, these girls' childhood whose pages had yellowed. The same ticks had simultaneously caused two very different clinical pictures in two sisters. The third sister had not been hospitalised at that time, but all three had ever since been more or less unwell into adulthood, and each one had developed her own autoimmune disease.

I treated Behçet's disease in the first of these sisters with antibiotics and hydroxychloroquine as classic treatments had failed (recurrent meningitis despite high doses of cortisone derivatives and colchicine). After an initial extremely violent exacerbation of symptoms that lasted for several weeks (excruciating pain requiring morphine and extreme drowsiness with sleep durations of 18 hours a day), she recovered within a few months and still has not relapsed 18 years after stopping treatment, except for occasional episodes of fatigue or discrete joint pain. I naively thought that this astounding medical story was going to spark the interest at least of my colleagues, but the comments from the reviewers of the medical journal who refused publication were so petty they were sad.

My experience with treating crypto-infections

Treatment is not a long, quiet river. As I accumulated experience over the years, I realised that I was improving 80% of my patients but the beneficial results were often not obvious at first and only 20% of patients recovered quickly.

As mentioned in earlier chapters, three quarters of patients go through long phases of their symptoms actually worsening (the Jarisch-Herxheimer of 'Herx' reaction), lasting from a few days to a few weeks, even a few months, before improving. Most often, the process is irregular, with phases of aggravation alternating with phases of improvement. This 'roller coaster' pattern (or 'yo-yoing' as I call these oscillations) may be observed over months. In the most common scenario, renewed onset of symptoms becomes less severe and less frequent before gradually disappearing. Unfortunately, many patients (and especially their family circle and/or their doctor) do not understand or accept this phenomenon and give up too soon. These aggravations or 'exacerbations' are sometimes extremely violent, giving the patient the impression that he or she is going to die. I know many who, despite being warned, have panicked and called paramedics. The usual result is that they wait for a few hours in an emergency department before ending up in psychiatry. After this exacerbation period, provided the same treatment is continued, many patients improve over time.

It is essential always to inform the patient and his or her relatives and doctor that exacerbations are very common and that, in some cases, they can be extremely violent. Fortunately, in most cases, they remain bearable, but it is better to prepare the patient for the worst. Most exacerbations do not put the patient at risk; it can be an unpleasant experience, but it will not last. I always advise patients never to introduce two new drugs or therapeutic plants on the same day because it can increase the reaction strength and then it is not known which product was involved. You should only add a second product after a few days, or even a few weeks, to be sure that the first is well tolerated. One must always keep in mind that an exacerbation may occur on the first day of treatment, sometimes within hours, but may be delayed by one, two, or even three weeks.

The usual reaction of a doctor when the patient suddenly gets worse after three weeks is to tell them: 'We are stopping everything. You can see clearly that the treatment is not working and that the infectious route is not the right one.' And yet, it is quite the opposite – it shows that it is working very well. I also recommend that patients who are working or students who are studying do not start a new treatment a few days before major professional meetings or exams. They may not be able to cope, and such failures can compromise their careers. Caution should be exercised in the following cases: epilepsy, depression, incomplete paralysis, severe eye problems and heart rhythm disorders. In the first few days, treatment can trigger an epileptic seizure (obviously dangerous while driving), aggravate depression with the risk of suicidal thinking, aggravate paralyses that become transitorily complete, cause a sudden worsening of vision, even transient blindness, or trigger a serious heart arrhythmia.

In all of these cases, I only start antibiotic treatment after the patient has seen his medical specialist for permission and to increase their anti-epileptic, antidepressant or antiarrhythmic treatment, for example. In case of severe eye damage, I ask the patient, after consulting his ophthalmologist, to carry steroids that can be taken in case of emergency to reduce eye inflammation. When these problems are anticipated, everything goes well. In the case of great anxiety on the part of the patient or the doctor, the treatment can be started at the hospital under close supervision.

I have rarely observed biological exacerbation reactions, but these are possible – that is, real biological 'herx' with, in particular, a rapid and strong rise of transaminase enzymes at the beginning of treatment. They go back down more or less quickly after the drug involved has been stopped. In cases where the patient has him/herself taken the same drug a little later on in the programme (which I would never have dared to prescribe because of the risks), I have been surprised to see that the transaminases have risen only weakly after reintroduction and then normalised, showing that this transient biological reaction was not related to a toxic effect of the drug.

For patients who have decreased lymphocytes before treatment begins, their numbers often drop slightly at the beginning of treatment and then rise again, sometimes months later. The increase in lymphocytes in the blood very often foreshadows clinical improvement and a significant reduction in symptoms. It's like primroses announcing the Spring.

The symptoms may disappear completely, but not everyone is so lucky, especially when the disease is of very longstanding. A background of irreducible symptoms may persist. Some feel almost completely cured but describe reappearance of their symptoms from time to time, which can last a few days. In women, the disease is often affected by the menstrual cycle, with menstrual flares. The condition often subsides during pregnancy but tends to explode after delivery. It may be that post-partum psychosis is the consequence of crypto-infections. If one settles for a simple antibiotic treatment for a few months, many patients recover or improve, but the huge problem is that at least 80% will relapse sooner or later. The relapse time after treatment is very variable, ranging from three days to three months or even three years. Severe stress, flu, surgery, a significant change in outside temperature or a new tick bite can trigger a relapse.

Some causes of failure

In my experience, complete failures of empiric antimicrobial treatments are rare, and these are probably related to other diseases or to the patients' attitude to their treatment. Some of these problem attitudes are as follows:

- The first is the patient who absolutely needs irrefutable proof of his diagnosis before deciding to accept treatment. In this case, I suggest that s/he comes back in 15 years to see if there is anything new to offer in the way of diagnostic tests!
- The second is the patient who refuses to accept getting worse before improving.
- The third is the patient who accepts the initial exacerbations, but who, after three yo-yos in the cyclical evolution of symptoms, breaks down and no longer believes in the diagnosis and the efficacy of treatment.
- The fourth is the patient whose family, medical or professional circle absolutely do not believe in chronic Lyme disease and constantly harass them so that they do not take their antimicrobial treatment and go to see a doctor elsewhere. I call these failures 'psycho-social-family-based'.
- The fifth is the patient living alone, especially with dependent children, who must work to put food on the table and run between work, the children's homework, shopping, day care and school. If treatments cause exacerbations that require long periods of rest, their lives become impossible and they stop all treatment. It is even worse when the spouse or the husband, family or in-laws call the patient lazy and/or a hypochoncriac and refuse to give any help. Looking back, many patients who have experienced this misunderstanding from those around them say that it is the most difficult thing to go through, often more difficult than the fatigue or permanent pain to which they can become accustomed.

How to treat crypto-infections in the absence of research

The 'therapeutic recipes' exchanged between 'crypto-infectiologists' around the world seem totally irrational from the outside, especially since doctors competent in the field cannot publish about their experience. Why is it that we use not only antibiotics that are active against *Borrelia*, but also various other antimicrobials, including antiparasitic and antifungal agents? These drugs probably work through their effectiveness against infections associated with *Borrelia*, especially parasites. These strategies are based on scientific work carried out in laboratories and, in some cases, on publications of clinical studies. In 2015, I published a review of medical articles on this subject in *La Presse Médicale*.[18] (This was the article so critised by the practitioner in Mulhouse.)

Antimalarial treatments

Several antimalarials are very effective in patients with chronic Lyme or related diseases: hydroxychloroquine (Plaquenil®), mefloquine (Lariam®), atovaquone-proguanil (Malarone®), artemisinin and especially *Artemisia annua*, the plant from which the drug is extracted. These antimalarial drugs often cause violent 'herx' reactions, wrongly said to be 'side effects' of the drug. But, as explained earlier, these exacerbations gradually disappear, to be followed by clear clinical improvement. It is highly likely to me that travellers who take preventive malaria treatments and suffer from 'adverse effects' are 'lymed' or 'crypto-infected'.

However, the most common side effect of antimalarials is mefloquine-induced depression. I remember the case of a young bride who went to the tropics for her honeymoon and who cried during her whole stay under the coconut trees. Caution should therefore be exercised in depressed patients, as mefloquine can induce suicidal thinking. In that case, psychiatric management is necessary before starting treatment for a crypto-infection.

In France and Belgium, a ban on marketing the plant *Artemisia annua* poses a real problem for some patients suffering from 'crypto-infections', because this plant often has a remarkable effect. This ban, still in existence in 2020, follows the death of a person suffering from malaria, who instead of consulting a doctor to be prescribed an artemisinin-based treatment (the chemical drug derived from the plant *Artemisia annua*), at the recommended dose for this potentially fatal disease, or another active and recommended drug, stupidly preferred to self-medicate by taking an insufficient dose. It is as though penicillin was banned because a patient died of a severe infection for self-medicating with an insufficient dose of that antibiotic. In fact, this case was a pretext. The pharmaceutical industry actively lobbies international bodies to ban the use of certain highly effective plants in order to protect the patent on the marketed chemical extract – in this case, artemisinin. For example, in Ireland, St John's wort is available only on prescription. Yet in traditional medicine, the whole plant *Artemisia* seems to be more active, works on other infections and does not induce resistance.

Hydroxychloroquine

In addition to its antiparasitic properties, which can act against *Babesiae* (other tick-borne micro-organisms), hydroxy-chloroquine has antibacterial properties, often unknown by physicians. Norwegian researchers have shown that this drug is directly active on *Borrelia burgdorferi*.[48] In addition, hydroxychloroquine contributes to the destruction of bacteria ingested by phagocytosis (that is, 'eaten' by white blood cells). Usually a bacterium is destroyed inside the white blood cells. However, so-called 'intracellular' bacteria can often survive and even multiply inside the white blood cell. This is the case, for example, with tuberculosis and Q fever. For these two bacterial diseases, hydroxychloroquine has been shown to promote the destruction of bacteria inside white blood cells. This effect considerably strengthens the effect of antibiotics. The same phenomenon has been observed with chronic Lyme disease.

However, note that hydroxychloroquine, even used alone, triggers an exacerbation of signs and symptoms that may be strong, three out of four times. That is why I always start this treatment in small doses (100 milligrammes per day for an adult) and only give a low dose in the long term (200 milligrammes per day) because this very powerful antimicrobial drug concentrates more than a thousand times in the small vesicles that contain the bacteria inside the white blood cell, the phagolysosomes. Curiously, this drug is widely used by general hospital physicians, rheumatologists, some dermatologists, neurologists and respiratory physicians to treat various autoimmune diseases. In the official version, this drug acts as an 'anti-inflammatory' or 'immunomodulator'. The official dose being high (two to three tablets of 200 milligrammes per day), half of the patients quickly stop the treatment because of 'side effects' which are actually poorly understood 'herx' reactions. Hydroxychloroquine also has antiviral effects. It has been shown that chloroquine and hydroxychloroquine were effective against the coronavirus responsible for SARS.[235, 197] Recently, with the Covid-19 pandemic, despite polemics, it has appeared according to several studies to be an effective treatment against the new coronavirus SARS-CoV-2, responsible for Covid-19.[26a, 58a, 58b, 64a, 124a]

I will not go into all the treatments here because, although they are effective, they are not validated by official research protocols. In some cases, they have been fortuitous discoveries by patients. Thus, a patient from Alsace, whom I saw regularly in consultation and who presented with chronic pains along the spine, called me one day to share her 'discovery'. Her grandchildren had caught pinworms, those little white worms you can see stirring in stools and that itch the anus. As she had been infected herself, she bought flubendazole (Fluvermal®), a well-known de-worming anti-parasitic drug, from her pharmacist. Usually for pinworms, a single tablet is sufficient, and it is then advised to take a second one after a space to avoid relapses. There are six tablets in the box. As she did not pay attention to the leaflet, she took one tablet a day for six days. She then noticed that, during this flubendazole treatment, her back and lumbar pain had clearly subsided. Off her own bat, without talking to her doctor, she took another six-day course of the drug from time to time and noticed that the signs of her chronic illness were fading away. When she told me of her finding, I was very doubtful because I could not find a plausible explanation. I told her that, if it allowed her to recover, I was not against her taking a course for a few days from time to time, but not more than once a month because, even if this drug seemed harmless and could be given to infants, there were no available data on its long-term use.

However, based on this information from my patient, when shortly after I saw another patient who had one of the most severe and rebellious forms of chronic Lyme I had had to treat and she asked me if there were any new avenues for treatment, I suggested she try flubendazole for six days to see if there was a reaction. She called me on the second day of taking the medication to tell me that it had caused an 'explosion' of her signs and symptoms of chronic Lyme. The multiple erythema migrans she had had 20 years earlier and her old knee arthritis, which had marked the beginning of her illness, had come back in full force as if by magic. I asked her to come immediately back to the hospital and I was able to see this re-emergence of enormous erythema migrans rashes and arthritis under the effect of a trivial de-worming medication. I biopsied an erythema migrans the same day in order to look for microbes but the analyses remained negative.

Since then, I have observed many times this effect of flubendazole which often causes exacerbations during the first treatment and then subsequently contributes to clinical improvement. I then remembered a child who had been cured of an acute form of Lyme disease on antibiotics and had relapsed a few months later in the days following a course of flubendazole his mother had given him because he had pinworms. This flubendazole effect is neither known nor studied. It is impossible to publish on the subject because parasitologists say it is impossible, especially since this drug is known to have little absorption into the body. And yet it works! I now share this experience of the benefits of flubendazole with many 'crypto-infectiologist' doctors in France and abroad.

My hypothesis is that residual bacteria that cause Lyme disease survive inside parasites and that an antiparasitic treatment makes the wolf come out of the woods. In the field of tropical medicine, these bacteria-parasite interactions are well-known, the most typical example being typhoid fever and schistosomiasis: *Salmonella typhi*, the bacterium responsible for typhoid fever, is capable of surviving antibiotic treatment in a patient by hiding in *Schistosomiae*, parasitic worms living in the blood of patients with schistosomiasis (bilharzia).

Apart from Lyme and related diseases, I have also seen that unexplained clinical condtions can react to antiparasitic trial treatment – for example, an African patient who was treated for tuberculosis had enlarged lymph nodes near the liver and right kidney that did not regress with anti-tuberculosis drugs. His right kidney had not been working at all for several months and its surgical removal was scheduled. As the abdominal ultrasound showed a thickening of the small intestine, it reminded me of a presentation compatible with digestive parasitosis though investigations did not reveal any parasites. In agreement with the patient, I tried out an antiparasitic drug, albendazole, before the kidney removal went ahead. What a surprise – three days after the beginning of the treatment, he started to urinate blood and then the right kidney started to function normally! He is now cured.

A few years ago, a farmer from the Pyrenees who had never travelled outside France presented with a severe form of Lyme disease, which was resistant to many of the treatments he had tried. For years he had had strange skin lesions with a thickening of the palms of his hands that cracked from time to time. He also had a benign unexplained cyst under his skin, facing a rib. He had consulted all the dermatologists in the region, including at the university hospital, but no one had been able to establish a diagnosis. He told me that he knew shepherds in his area who had the same lesions. As he had already received many antibiotics, I wondered if it could be a parasitosis. I suggested a short course of various antiparasitic drugs to him, including a four-day treatment with ivermectin.

While taking this drug, normally intended to treat tropical parasitic infections, he went through an extremely violent exacerbation reaction of all his symptoms, including diffuse pain and fatigue. He was bedridden by the reaction. The cyst that was palpable under the skin became painful and doubled in volume. I asked him to have it removed for analysis, but nothing was found in it. In the days that followed the course of ivermectin, he felt in very good shape and the skin lesions on his hands disappeared. Unfortunately, he relapsed a few weeks later, apart from his skin lesions, which returned only occasionally in a very attenuated form. Since then and for several years now, he has been taking a four-day course of ivermectin from time to time, because it is one of the rare drugs that allows him to cope in the long term.

This intermittent intake of a few days of active medication is part of the strategy in the maintenance phase of chronic Lyme disease treatment. Sequential treatments of different drugs are often used, given in small courses of a few days each, in rotation. Some antibiotics also have antiparasitic properties, such as metronidazole and tinidazole, which are also very active on persistent round forms of *Borrelia*. Antifungals are often effective, such as fluconazole and griseofulvin. The effectiveness of fluconazole against persistent forms of *Borrelia burgdorferi* was demonstrated in 2015 in the laboratory by Zhang and collaborators.[87] It is reassuring that this antimicrobial activity has now been shown in vitro (in the lab), because 'crypto-infectiologists' have been using this drug for years in the treatment of chronic Lyme disease. Initially, it was a German doctor, himself seriously ill with paralysis, who, after taking a lot of antibiotics, developed oral candidiasis, or 'thrush'. He took fluconazole as an antifungal active against *Candida albicans* and to his great surprise, the drug improved his condition and he was able to get out of his wheelchair.

A clinical study was conducted and published in 2004 by Schardt showing the benefit of fluconazole in the treatment of chronic Lyme.[198] I was always surprised to see that all imidazole derivatives, whether antibacterial, antiparasitic or antifungal, could have a beneficial effect on patients. When all goes well, in the majority of cases, these sequential non-antibiotic treatments can be continued a few days a month for a few months. This prevents possible long-term toxicity and contributes to avoiding bacterial resistance.

Some patients have Lyme disease that mimicks a typical autoimmune disease. One of my colleagues confessed to seeing a young man with multiple sclerosis recover with prolonged antibiotic treatment over several months. His dermatologist had prescribed a small dose of doxycycline long-term for acne. Acne treatment cured his multiple sclerosis! Lyme antimicrobial treatment sometimes completely cures the autoimmune disease, but quite often this treatment brings about an incomplete improvement. This suggests that there are other factors also mainaining the disease. These could be viruses for which we currently have no treatment or other genetic, inflammatory or autoimmune factors.

It has been published that the plaques seen in the brain or spinal cord of patients with multiple sclerosis contain the sixth herpes virus, HHV-6.[132] A recent publication has also shown a link between multiple sclerosis and the presence of a variant of the Epstein-Barr virus, the agent causing infectious mononucleosis ('glandular fever').[148] In complicated cases of autoimmune disease, the best results can be obtained when one can work intelligently and synergistically with the disease specialist (a neurologist in the case of multiple sclerosis, a rheumatologist in the case of rheumatoid arthritis, etc) who can suggest new active treatments on some disease processes. The anti-infective approach with the 'crypto-infections' hypothesis should not be opposed to the classical approach which tackles the disease from another angle, including with immunosuppressants when there is no choice. This applies to all medical specialties but requires an open mind on the part of the specialist physician. I would like to salute Professor Olivier Lyon-Caen, an eminent neurologist specialising in multiple sclerosis at the Pitié-Salpêtrière Hospital, because he is one of the rare specialty professors to raise such questions. From time to time he would send me patients for consultation when he was hesitating between Lyme and multiple sclerosis.

The role of the environment and ticks in the genesis of crypto-infections

Now that I have accumulated considerable experience with many autoimmune diseases and with Lyme disease, I systematically look for a possible vector exposure. I have seen lupus, rheumatoid arthritis, multiple sclerosis, etc, start after camping, a scout camp, a hike or lily of the valley or mushroom picking. I observe many thyroid pathologies in patients with chronic

Lyme disease. I have wondered if the large number of people who complained of thyroiditis, or even thyroid cancer, after eating mushrooms gathered in the forest and who pointed to the radioactive cloud of Chernobyl as the culprit did not rather have Lyme or another crypto-infection caught from ticks during numerous ventures into the forest.

A patient had contracted a very severe case of Still's disease after a walk in the forest, which I had cured with antimicrobials. I had warned him against ticks, but three years later, on a holiday in the Vosges forest, he could not resist swimming in a lake in the middle of the forest. The place was apparently magnificent with a natural waterfall and ferns shining in the sun. Fifteen days after this escapade, he relapsed with again all the signs and symptoms of serious Still's disease.

One day I saw a patient who wanted to sue a great Parisian medical professor who was treating her for lupus. She was shocked with hindsight because this doctor had not asked her the circumstances of its beginning. She had had a tick bite in her navel, later surrounded by an erythema migrans, before developing lupus.

Happy pachyderms

I dream of having hard skin, not only to resist the attacks of anti-chronic Lyme people, but also because of our tick friends. All animals that live in nature are affected by tick-borne diseases and age prematurely, becoming rheumatic. Even the lion, the king of animals, ends up tired, loses his hair and his libido and struggles to run eventually. Perhaps it will change the day lions are treated with herbal medicine and surgeons give them hip prostheses made of antelope bone! Who lives 100 years in the wild? Thick-skinned animals: elephants, rhinos, etc. Yet ticks are found on them and tick-borne diseases are reported. But perhaps their tough skin reduces the risks.

Animals have other defences. A widespread Californian lizard is a very common prey for tick nymphs. The blood of this lizard contains a protein capable of killing *Borrelia*. As a result, adult lizards are very rarely infected. Remember always to have a Californian lizard with you!

Chronic unexplained syndromes that start after serious infections

In addition to chronic syndromes that typically appear after chronic viral infections or infections that are capable of becoming chronic, such as EBV and cytomegalovirus (CMV), or linked to hepatitis B or C viruses, it now appears that comparable chronic syndromes may appear after various acute infections that are not known to be persistent. These chronic syndromes usually combine severe fatigue and fibromyalgia with muscle or joint pain and, in some cases, manifestations resembling various autoimmune disorders. This is sometimes seen after legionellosis. There is a group of legionellosis victims whose members complain of serious and persistent health concerns following the acute illness. More recently, a large number of syndromes of the same type have been observed after recovery from acute diseases such as chikungunya ('Chik') and Ebola.

My hypothesis is that crypto-infections that are quietly dormant in the individual can wake up during an acute infectious illness. It is interesting to note that, according to our colleagues on Réunion Island, hydroxychloroquine, a powerful broad-spectrum antimicrobial as I have explained above, has proved effective in many cases of chronic post-Chik syndrome. I was sorry that our rheumatologist and general medicine colleagues preferred to use methotrexate, an immunosuppressant, to treat these post-Chik syndromes. Their reason was that they observed excerbations of signs and symptoms with hydroxychloroquine. These exacerbations are probably 'Herx' phenomena, since they disappear after a bit even if treatment is maintained. These excarbations were considered to be 'side effects' by many physicians.

In Garches, where many victims of polio in France in the 1950s and early 1960s were treated, my neurological physiotherapist colleagues have found many cases of 'post-polio syndrome'. These are people who had recovered from the infection but retained residual paralysis and whose paralysis reactivated with aging, decades later. The cause is unknown. Could crypto-infections that develop with age be the cause?

In 2020, many patients worldwide who developed Covid-19 infection and recovered from their acute disease, subsequently complained of persistent signs and symptoms similar to chronic Lyme disease. I'm convinced that crypto-infections are, at least partially, involved in these 'post-Covid' syndromes. This hypothesis should be studied in research protocols. The only vision of many of my colleagues is that these problems are purely psychosomatic!

Not everything is due to ticks

Silent co-infections by microbes not transmitted by ticks are also likely. For example, at least 50% of French people, who love to eat red meat and steak tartare, harbour toxoplasma *(Toxoplasma gondii)* for life in their nervous system, including their brain, and muscles in particular, while only 22% of Americans, who usually eat their meat well done, harbour these charming parasites in their brains. The frequency is higher than 90% in some developing countries. That said, as we are becoming more American in our eating habits, the frequency of toxoplasmosis is decreasing among young French people. We can't have it all, obesity and toxoplasmosis! It is usually said that toxoplasma is dormant and has no consequences (except in pregnant women, because of the congenital infection that attacks the foetus), but what do we really know? If deep immunosuppression occurs, toxoplasmosis can wake up and cause serious complications.

Very sadly, toxoplasma brain abscesses were seen daily during the AIDS epidemic, before the development of effective antiretroviral triple therapies. Two recent Swedish publications show that, in healthy subjects, being infected with toxoplasma increases the risk of suicide attempts sevenfold.[175, 245] This does not mean that toxoplasma is the agent of suicide, but it probably reflects that toxoplasma, during its survival cycles, contributes to an episodic inflammation or a temporary disruption of certain functions in the nervous system with other factors and that, if one has other reasons to want to commit suicide, it promotes that thinking.

Among bacterial infections, *Coxiella burnetii* (the agent of Q fever) is a well-known example of an infection that can become chronic and cause serious health problems, including heart-valve damage. This bacterium, mainly present in the placenta of infected animals, especially domestic sheep, goats and cattle, is transmitted to humans mainly by the inhalation of contaminated dust or manure, more rarely by tick bites. In cases of strong winds, the spores of *Coxiella* can be transmitted miles away. The Netherlands, a very windy country, has painfully experienced this after they massively developed factory-farms crowding together thousands of animals. People who live downwind of these farms have experienced Q fever outbreaks. That will create a lot of work for heart surgeons in a few years.

In the south of France, a large part of the population is sheltering *Leishmaniae*, protozoan parasites transmitted by a biting midge, the blackfly. The parasites mainly infect dogs in the region from Montpellier to Nice via Marseille. Most infected people are not sick. There again, during the AIDS epidemic, we regularly saw patients with severe leishmaniasis, because immunosuppression allowed the parasites to wake up. Are these *Leishmaniae* asleep all the time in everyone?

Some viruses that are widespread in the population remain in the body for life after the initial infection. It is so for the herpes viruses known as simplex (HHV-1 and HHV-2), the varicella virus that can wake up by giving shingles (varicella-zoster virus, VZV), the Epstein-Barr virus (EBV – the agent of infectious mononucleosis), cytomegalovirus (CMV) and the sixth human herpes virus (HHV-6). Under certain circumstances, some of these viruses may be involved in chronic diseases in humans.

It is known that primary EBV and CMV infection both greatly weaken the immune system for a limited period of time, and that this can sometimes be the starting point for chronic diseases. EBV, when caught in the first year of life by babies living in Africa in some areas heavily contaminated with malaria, induces a form of cancer, Burkitt's lymphoma. This example shows that very different microbes can form 'criminal associations' to trigger or maintain serious diseases, including cancer. Moreover, during infectious mononucleosis due to EBV, it is better, unless one wants to scare onself, not to remove or biopsy the lymph nodes which often become very large during this disease – under a microscope, the presence of Sternberg cells, characteristic of the malignant lymphoma, Hodgkin's disease, can be observed in the mononucleosis ganglia.

The brain plaques of multiple sclerosis patients are often filled with HHV-6 inclusions. Is this virus a cofactor in the disease? Neurologists usually say the opposite: that HHV-6 fixes itself on the plaques because of local tissue disturbances, but that it is only passing through without being involved and that the viruses stopped there because there was some inflammation. This reminds me of gastroenterologists' comments about *Helicobacter pylori* in stomach ulcers or *Mycobacterium avium subspecies paratuberculosis* in Crohn's disease lesions (see page 186).

The VZV virus, responsible for chickenpox, persists in the body throughout life and may wake up in some people to cause shingles. This virus can persist in our arteries. For example, rare cases of stroke are observed during shingles adjacent to the carotid artery. This VZV virus has also been suspected by Gilden of promoting the onset of giant cell temporal arteritis, known as Horton's disease.[98]

We know that mycobacteria, particularly tuberculosis bacilli, can persist in our arteries and their role has also been suspected in Horton's disease, as well as in a very severe vasculitis that can affect the aorta, Takayasu's disease. I remember a woman who had had an aorta operation for Takayasu's disease and whose arterial wall was filled with tubercle bacilli under the microscope. There was, at one time, a lot of enthusiasm for the bacterial cause of atherosclerosis, which is responsible, in particular, for myocardial infarction. The bacterium *Chlamydia pneumoniae*, usually responsible for acute pneumonia, has been implicated and chronic carriage in the bronchi may be an important factor in chronic asthma in children. When this bacterium is injected intravenously into some animals, they rapidly develop atheroma plaques in their arteries. Some treatment trials of astherosclerosis by antibiotic have been conducted but were inconclusive. Indeed, it seems unlikely that an antibiotic used alone for limited periods would have a chance of reducing old atheroma plaques, stuffed with biofilms.

However, it has been shown in animals that an antibiotic, doxycycline, prevents the formation of aortic aneurysms and can reduce their progression. An aneurysm corresponds to an abnormal dilatation of the artery, in consequence of a weakening of its wall due to atheroma lesions. The risk is aneurysm rupture which is often fatal. A Dutch study, published by Arnoud-Meyer in 2013, tested patients who already had small aortic aneurysms.[27] They compared doxycycline to placebo and concluded that doxycycline was ineffective. However, when we look closely at the results, we realise that doxycycline, unlike a placebo, caused a moderate increase in aneurysm size during the study with highly significant statistical test results. This means that doxycycline triggered an inflammatory reaction in the arterial wall, presumably linked to an exacerbation caused by the destruction of bacteria residing there. Fluoroquinolones are antibiotics which may worsen some aneurysms, probably, at least in part, as a result of the same phenomenon.

The hepatitis viruses

Chronic infections with the hepatitis B virus can lead to autoimmune diseases, the most famous being periarteritis nodosa (PAN). I do not treat patients with PAN because it is often a serious disease requiring highly specialised management, but I have wondered about it when seeing certain patients. The rare few I have seen with the condition had been multiply exposed to nature and on two occasions I suspected associated parasitosis. I prescribed an antiparasitic (albendazole) for a few days, and they had very violent general exacerbation reactions, with fever at 40°C and massive sweating. It would not surprise me if parasites were involved in some forms of this disease.

During my senior registrar period in the 1980s, the hepatitis C virus was not yet known and the term 'non-A non-B hepatitis' was used. At the same time, general physicians were looking after many patients presenting with an 'idiopathic' autoimmune disease. This was a form of 'cryoglobulinaemia' that was treated without much success with immunosuppressants. When the hepatitis C virus (HCV) was discovered and a blood test was developed for it, it was quickly realised that these cryoglobulinaemias were not falling from the sky but were indeed a complication of hepatitis C. 'Idiopathic cryoglobulinaemia' disappeared after effective treatment of hepatitis C with antivirals. I am always happy when a disease goes from the 'idiopathic' to the 'infectious' box because it often changes the deal for the patient.

Gut diseases and antimicrobial treatments

When I was a surgery student in Paris in 1975, there were still old-fashioned nightingale wards shared by up to 40 patients.

Surgeons made their rounds sporting a large apron and about 20 people – wardens, nurses, students, medical trainees – religiously followed the visit. In all departments at the time, the chief nurse, like Saint Peter, had a large set of keys, a sign of her absolute power and had the heavy responsibility of preparing the plastic fingerstall and the Vaseline for the sacrosanct digital rectal examination to which all patients were subjected. These patients had already had at least 10 rectal examinations from all the students and housemen, but the examination by the senior registrar was a supreme act that was looked at with respect. All the patients in the surrounding beds were at the show. I remember a poor traumatised young woman curling up at the top of her bed. She had Whipple's disease, a chronic multivisceral disease, often affecting the intestine, which at the time was 'idiopathic' and often considered 'psychosomatic' because of the frequency of neurological disorders and psychological repercussions. However, since the 1950s some doctors had observed that these patients could be improved, or even cured, with antibiotics. However, many surgeons treated patients by intestinal resection in the event of digestive complications.

Once the triumphant index finger was stuck in the young woman's buttocks, I can still hear this surgeon declaiming loudly to the whole ward, in front of the terrified woman: 'Gentlemen, Whipple's disease is a form of hysteria that must be surgically excised!'

At the time, Crohn's disease was also often considered 'hysterical'. I have seen the same behaviours in front of sick women with scarred abdomens from multiple operations in the management of this disease. Fortunately, the head of the department, an eminent professor of surgery, was very humane with his patients, but he did not control everything in his department.

Nowadays, we know that Whipple's disease is an infectious disease, for which the responsible bacterium, *Tropheryma whipplei*, has been isolated, and which can be cured with antibiotics. These cases remind me of a more recent episode in Garches where a woman with fibromyalgia was hospitalised for chronic Lyme disease. As I walked down the corridor, I crossed paths with a visiting psychiatrist coming out of her room. He was explaining, very proudly, in front of the students, the residents and the nurse: 'Fibromyalgia is the hysteria of modern times!' This shows that old habits die hard.

Multiple routes of transmission of infectious diseases

There are many ways in which microbes enter the body (airborne, digestive, transcutaneous, sexual, transplacental, by injection, by contact with some mucous membranes, various and varied animal vectors, etc). Even for a vector-borne disease such as Lyme, essentially transmitted by tick bites, other modes of contamination are possible. Indeed, cases of transmission by other vectors have been reported or suspected. I once saw a model posing for a fashion shoot at Iguaçu Falls at the border of Brazil and Argentina develop multiple erythema migrans rashes at the site of each mosquito bite she received. But mosquitoes seem to be bad vectors. A few people have got sick after being bitten by chiggers. Spiders, horseflies and lice have also been mentioned.

Chickens are excellent tick predators and they can rid your garden of them, but this is not always without risk. Beware of the poultry red mite! I was consulted by a Belgian couple living in the suburbs of Brussels with their 4-year-old daughter. Everyone had been in perfect health until the day they had decided to raise some chickens in their garden. After a short interval the mother and daughter started getting terrible itching, then fell seriously ill with outbreaks of fever associated with a whole set of pains and neurological signs. The little girl, who had always been happy, changed character, often crying, and suffered from terrible nightmares. Then they realised that red mites were running all over their bodies and that there were plenty in the henhouse.

Red mites are small vampires that can be found in poultry houses as well as dovecotes. They attack sleeping animals at night, suck their blood, then withdraw again. The father, who was more resistant, did not get sick. The doctors, as they could not understand anything about these symptoms and found no biological abnormalities, attributed all this to psychiatric problems. All the blood tests were negative. Fortunately, a Belgian doctor who was perfectly familiar with Lyme disease had an Elispot performed (the test described in Chapter 7, page 120, that is commonly performed in Germany but not recognised in France or Belgium); this was very positive for Lyme disease.

Lyme disease can also be transmitted through other routes. Transplacental transmission (from mother to baby in utero) is known and sexual, breastfeeding and transfusion transmissions are likely, but these have not yet been properly evaluated. In 2018, materno-foetal transmission of Lyme disease was recognised by the World Health Organization (International Classification of Diseases 11 – ICD11), but this recognition was withdrawn in December 2018 after lobbying by Canadian public health officials. Fortunately for the population, it is very likely that many people are healthy carriers of the *Borreliae* that cause Lyme disease, and also of other crypto-infections. A recent study published by Aase found *Borrelia* in the blood of healthy people.[20] These asymptomatic infected people are not sick and naturally control their infection. However, with other examples of latent infectious diseases, such as tuberculosis, it is known that a dormant infection can wake up and cause illness when circumstances change.

Cancer and crypto-infections

Doctors who treat chronic Lyme have all seen disturbingly plausible links between chronic infection and malignant lymphoma or cancer. This link is known for some viruses, but bacterial and parasitic leads are investigated less. In lymph nodes, tissue lesions are very similar, sometimes almost identical, between 'cat scratch disease' caused by *Bartonella* bacteria and malignant lymphomas such as Hodgkin's disease. Bacterial causes have been identified in some lymphomas. In 2001, with Ghez, we published a disturbing story. A 40-year-old man was hospitalised with an unexplained high fever of 39°C for at least three weeks.[6] Scanning had found a typical image of spleen lymphoma, a malignant disease that is treated by removal of the spleen and heavy cancer chemotherapy. As the radiological diagnosis was certain, contact had been made with a great Parisian haematology department, and the haematologists told us that this clinical situation was serious and that it was necessary to treat his lymphoma quickly and aggressively.

The patient was to be transferred early the following week. The removal of his spleen was scheduled at the same time as a bone marrow biopsy to look for a spread of his lymphatic cancer. Anti-cancer induction chemotherapy was scheduled in a second phase. It was Friday evening and I stayed with the patient to talk with him and cheer him up before the terrible ordeal that awaited him. I questioned him again to make sure I hadn't missed any other clues. I looked again for contact with vectors or animals. The patient then had a light-bulb moment and told me he remembered being scratched by a kitten a few weeks earlier. As I did not want to let any possible infectious cause pass, I decided with a collaborator, in agreement with the patient, to try a test antibiotic treatment over the weekend. On the Monday morning, the patient was all smiles and the fever had clearly regressed. I rushed to cancel the haematology transfer. Confirmation of an infectious cause was subsequently obtained because the result of blood tests always takes a while to come back. This was an exceptional clinical presentation of cat scratch disease caused by *Bartonella henselae*.

I also remember two patients with intermittent fever and with a multiple-organ syndrome that had been explored from every angle. An antimicrobial test treatment was attempted. After a few phases of initial worsening with the treatment, the patients began to feel much better and considered themselves recovered. They no longer had a fever and were gaining weight. During a mild flare-up of symptoms during treatment, as is common, small lymph nodes appeared. The biopsy showed some lymphoma-like cells. I then had to hand over to the haematologists. In both cases, the patients died a few months later of complications from chemotherapy. These observations left a bitter taste in my mouth because I was deeply convinced that their history was infectious and that they were getting better before the change of course. I very much regretted the lack of reliable diagnostic tests on this occasion.

Helicobacter pylori, the bacterium responsible for gastric and duodenal peptic ulcer disease, is now recognised as a carcinogenic bacterium. In 1994, the WHO classified *it* as a gastric carcinogen. In addition to stomach adenocarcinomas, this bacterium is also responsible for gastric lymphoma, called MALT, as published by Delchier in 2003.[67] Parisian colleagues with Marc Lecuit also showed the link between a cousin of *Helicobacter pylori*, *Campylobacter jejuni*, and an immunoproliferative disease of the small intestine.

I have also seen definite Lyme disease cases treated with cancer chemotherapy for 'malignant lymphoma'. If one has the misfortune of having a biopsy on an erythema migrans or a borrelian lymphocytoma (a small red ball on the ear, nipple or scrotum) which are characteristic skin manifestations of Lyme disease, it is well known and published that one can observe an appearance identical to that of malignant lymphoma on tissue analysis. Yet these lesions heal well with antibiotics. I have several times observed patients who were looked after by renowned medical teams that had not even thought of Lyme and who had very quickly found themselves in anti-cancer chemotherapy. Fortunately, they survived this ordeal, but relapsed from their Lyme sometime later. I was able to cure them subsequently with an antimicrobial treatment.

I have also experienced similar situations several times in my career with tuberculosis. Tuberculosis lesions can in some cases look deceptively like cancer. Thus, I have seen people have their vocal cord, uterus, bowel, kidney or complete lymph node chains removed before the doctor realised too late that it was a perfectly curable infectious disease. I was almost fooled in my department about 15 years ago when a handicapped girl was hospitalised for an acute case of an incomplete bowel obstruction with peritonitis. The surgeon called me immediately after coming out of the operating room to tell me that he had observed a picture typical of peritoneal carcinosis, which included the classic 'candle stains' appearance characteristic of cancer metastasised to the peritoneum, the envelope of the intestines. He had closed the patient up without performing any surgery (after the fact, I blessed him for not performing intestinal or other organ ablations), thinking that the situation was desperate in the very short term. I found it very surprising that a cancer hitherto unknown in this young girl could give such large scattered lesions in a short space of time. Fortunately, analysis of the surgical biopsies showed that the problem actually was intestinal and peritoneal tuberculosis. The infection was cured with anti-tuberculosis treatment.

These examples show that the link between chronic infections and cancers is not simple and can confuse doctors in their diagnostic process. I am convinced that cells in our body that are 'inhabited' in the long term by certain microbes can become cancerous. Some cancers, stomach cancer in particular, have decreased significantly since the introduction of antibiotics. Before the era of antibiotics, doctors often observed inoperable chronic bone infections. The infected area naturally drained through the skin through a path, called a fistula, which pus had dug through the muscle and subcutaneous tissue. Some war casualties thus 'leaked' for decades with a daily emission of pus. They preferred that to amputation, and we understand them. Some developed cancer around the fistula pathway after years, demonstrating the carcinogenic potential of chronic infection.

Neoehrlichia mikurensis, a bacterium transmitted by ticks and which is beginning to be isolated in humans in various countries (except France...), can cause diseases of an autoimmune appearance but is also found in lesions similar to those of malignant lymphomas. This bacterium is present in French ticks, but no reliable diagnostic test has been developed to detect it, not only in my country, but also not in Great Britain or the rest of Europe.

Recently, researchers have shown that a parasite responsible for a condition called piroplasmosis in animals, close to *Babesiae*, called *Theileria*, transmitted by ticks and present in cattle, sheep, goats and horses, is capable of transforming a healthy human cell into a cancerous one and that the process is reversible. In animals, *Theileriae* are known to cause malignant lymphomas. This would merit further research on parasites of the genus *Theileria*. Over the years, one notices that ticks are not insignificant and are perhaps responsible for many more health problems than we believe today.

Meanwhile, gums damaged by paradontitis and rotten teeth are not only a factor promoting Alzheimer's (see page 197), but also oesophageal cancer. The link between a dental plaque bacterium, *Porphyromonas gingivalis*, and oesophageal cancer has recently been discovered. This work, published by Gao in 2016,[94] was carried out by the University of Louisville School of Dentistry in the United States in collaboration with a Chinese team. As we have seen above (page 197), *Porphyromonas gingivalis* has also been found in the brains of Alzheimer's patients, as have *Borrelia* and *Treponema* spirochetes.

Perhaps crypto-infections could also explain the inflammatory manifestations that come with some cancers. These signs and symptoms are called 'para-neoplastic syndromes'. They can cause neurological, hormonal, blood, skin, bone and joint disorders. These manifestations, which have not been satisfactorily explained so far, occur at a distance from the cancerous tumour and do not contain malignant cells.

In 2015, Feng and Sharma showed that certain anticancer drugs have proved to be powerful antibiotics, active in particular on *Borrelia burgdorferi*.[86] To drive the message home, the effectiveness of other antibiotics has also been shown experimentally in various cancer models and on different forms of cancerous cell. In a recent study, it was shown that antibiotics that act on mitochondria (the organelles in all animal cells that produce energy by metabolising oxygen and originated as bacteria) were capable of eradicating cancer stem cells. In 2015, Lamb and his colleagues suggested changing the approach to cancer and treating it as an infectious disease.[125]

The supposed 'anti-inflammatory' effect of some antibiotics

When publications are released on the effects of antibiotics on some chronic inflammatory diseases, the possible 'anti-inflammatory' or 'immunomodulatory' effect of antibiotics is most often highlighted. These anti-inflammatory effects have been described with various classes of antibiotics, including tetracyclines and macrolides. As though by chance, these antibiotics are those that work well on intracellular microbes. It is highly likely that the sometimes-dramatic action of these antibiotics in these situations is due to direct antimicrobial action on crypto-infections responsible for the inflammation and not this hypothetical anti-inflammatory effect that has most of the time only been studied in vitro on artificial models. In these experiments, antibiotics in high doses were used in the presence of immune cells to measure the variation in the production of this or that molecule usually produced by this cell.

Similarly, I have never fully comprehended why, in chronic obstructive bronchitis, antibiotics ineffective on bacteria found in sputum culture, are still active on the disease. This efficacy has even been observed against a placebo. I am convinced that, in this disease, the bronchial tubes contain invisible intracellular microbes that maintain the inflammatory process of the bronchial tubes over the years. *Haemophilus influenzae* is able to persist chronically, but there are surely others. In addition to inhaled pollutants, this could also explain obstructive pulmonary disease in people who do not smoke. Similarly, studies have shown that, for the treatment of pneumococcal pneumonia, the efficacy of the treatment was better, as was the prognosis, if the usual antibiotic active on the *Pneumococcus* (amoxicillin or ceftriaxone) was combined with another antibiotic active on intracellular bacteria (macrolide or fluoroquinolone). The very surprising part is that this beneficial effect is maintained if the *Pneumococcus* is resistant to the second intracellular antibiotic. My hypothesis is that people with severe pneumococcal pneumonia have lungs that at baseline are latently affected by crypto-infections that will contribute to aggravation during acute pneumococcal infection.

Interestingly, prolonged antibiotic therapies, sometimes lasting for more than a year, are used in certain specialties, such as respiratory medicine and rheumatology. A patient who presents with chronic inflammatory rheumatoid arthritis may be diagnosed with 'seronegative rheumatoid arthritis' (as explained earlier, that is without the rheumatoid factor, the classic marker of the disease, being found) if s/he consults a rheumatologist and may be diagnosed with 'seronegative Lyme disease' if he comes to see me. If the rheumatologist diagnoses seronegative polyarthritis without any evidence, he is said to be a great clinician. If, in addition, he prescribes one or two years of doxycycline, minocycline, clarithromycin or levofloxacin 'for anti-inflammatory purposes', this does not shock anyone, does not upset health insurance, and this practitioner is considered to be a great innovator.

However, seronegative rheumatoid arthritis is an 'expert diagnosis' that can lead to giving months of antibiotics without proof. If another doctor (maybe me...) prescribes four months of doxycycline to kill *Borrelia* and maybe some co-infections, it makes 'experts' protest, and say it is a scandal to treat Lyme disease without evidence beyond the officially recommended period with a drug that can cause bacterial resistance. If the latter doctor is a general practitioner, s/he risks going before a disciplinary board. I would like someone to explain to me why an antibiotic, when given as a possible 'anti-inflammatory', would not cause resistance? These surely are double standards. Similar are the very prolonged prescriptions of doxycycline to treat acne. This treatment is officially recognised. It is very common to see teenagers and young adults take this antibiotic for months and even years without anyone worrying or upsetting the authorities.

During the HIV-AIDS epidemic, before the advent of antiretroviral triple therapies, millions of people worldwide were continuously treated for life with daily antibiotic therapy, most often with a sulphonamide, but also with other antibiotics and/or other antimicrobials. It never occurred to anyone to yell blue murder.

Chapter 10

When medical methodology replaces medicine

The methodologies for identifying diseases and their causes, and for evaluating their treatments, have to meet objective criteria. However, often these methodologies have been developed in relatively simple situations with a limited number of parameters; these methods are totally inappropriate for the assessment of complex multi-factorial situations such as Lyme disease and 'crypto-infections' where an impressive number of different factors tend to interconnect. Reductive approaches, imposed by modern methodologies, lead to overlooking a whole set of factors. These symptomatic pictures, so complex and far from stereotypical, require other approaches that are no less objective but different, to be identified, understood and treated. The widely accepted methods have become an 'epistemological barrier' to understanding crypto-infections.

The over-reliance on randomised studies

When I was a medical student, I remember a lecture in a university amphitheatre at Beaujon Hospital in Clichy, France. A great medical professor spoke to us about research methods. He explained to us (it was in the 1970s) that, in Anglo-Saxon countries, researchers used amoral practices and drew lots to suggest different treatments, even the use of a fake drug called a placebo.

He told us of sinister episodes in the United States where mentally ill adults or children, poor black people and prisoners had been used as guinea pigs. These facts are now well-known and at least 40 studies of this type have been officially counted in the United States or abroad (the largest of them was conducted in Guatemala). The US Prison Service only banned these practices in prisons in the mid-1970s. As the pharmaceutical industry always needs people for experimentation, the practice then evolved towards asking patients to sign an 'informed consent' form before participating in trials.

Our teacher then told us: 'Rest assured, this kind of practice will never come to France, where scientists are humanists, deeply imbued with Ancient Greek and Latin culture'. In fact, randomised studies were beginning to take place in France in haematology and oncology under the impetus of drug manufacturers. They did not yet exist in the field of infectious diseases. The most well-regarded randomised studies are those where neither the patient nor the physician knows what is in the tablet or vial. These trials are called 'double-blind' randomised trials.

It was with the appearance of AIDS that this methodology was first used in France for infectious diseases. Shortly after the beginning of my work as a senior registrar in 1985, the development of the first therapeutic trials of drugs for AIDS began. A drug, suramin, had been proposed (which would prove ineffective against HIV). I remember a heated discussion in the INSERM research building located in the old Claude-Bernard Hospital, where a dozen experts sitting around the table were tearing each other apart to decide whether a placebo should be used and, if so, whether patients should be told that they might receive a fake medication. Opinions were very divided. Could we ethically tell someone we knew was condemned to death by an illness that we were going to draw lots and that the treatment we were going to try on them and that they were putting all of their hope on might not work or might be a placebo?

We must not forget that at the time, in France, cancer patients were not told their diagnosis. Fortunately, this has changed a lot, especially thanks to the appearance of more effective treatments, even if they are not always completely effective. Since that period, French research, but also global research, has drawn up standards for conducting randomised trials, including getting informed consent from patients. In general, the adoption of this norm has enabled great progress in the transparency of research and patient empowerment. However, in practice, understanding and acceptance by patients depends very much on the cultural context conditioning the perception of the disease and the physician, as you will see later (page 239).

The limitations of randomised studies

Apart from these cultural considerations, which are nevertheless fundamental, the medical limitations of randomised studies must be emphasised. The methodology is far from perfect; it is best used to answer a simple question, by varying only one factor (for example, an antibiotic or placebo) in a homogeneous population of patients for whom there are easily measurable objective signs. Unfortunately, this methodological approach is totally unsuitable when one has to study several interrelated factors, all the more so when the population of patients being studied is heterogeneous. A randomised study looking at only one placebo-controlled factor often requires a few hundred patients and around one million pounds. If two factors vary, we need thousands of patients and tens, even hundreds of millions, of pounds. In other words, it is impossible to evaluate. Only a few very promising molecules from the pharmaceutical industry are the subject of such trials, because the manufacturer is hoping to see a 'return on investment'. The problem with current clinical research and misunderstood evidence-based medicine is that everything that is not demonstrated by drawing lots ceases to exists. The insistence on 'all randomised double-blind' trials has the effect of abusing the medical community, and in some cases prevents any initiative and any advance in medicine.

Some cheap old medicines that have worked very well for decades have been tossed onto the garbage heap of history on the pretext that they have not been subjected to this methodology. For example, griseofulvin, an old antifungal that worked very well in some cases of lupus and that once appeared in *Le Dictionnaire Vidal des Médicaments* (France's main drug registry) with this official indication: 'adjunctive treatment of lupus', was moved a few years later to the status of: 'use with caution in case of lupus because it can cause flare-ups of symptoms', then more recently under the heading 'contraindicated in lupus'. Indeed, griseofulvin, which is a powerful antimicrobial, can cause exacerbations in the early treatment of lupus and of Lyme disease. However, patients with chronic Lyme disease often improve, after an initial aggravation phase, with small doses of griseofulvin.

In the early 1980s, 'experts' questioned the anti-aggregating properties of aspirin on blood platelets – small blood cells responsible for clot formation. When I was a medical resident, I read with dismay in a major international medical journal that American 'researchers' were getting informed consent from people who were going to have surgery on their lefthand heart chambers for various reasons so that the right side of their hearts could also be opened (which was not at all necessary for their treatment) in order to cut off the end of the catheter located there for analysis. (When you have heart surgery, they always put a tube, called a catheter, through the veins into the right chambers of the heart to infuse fluids and make recordings.) The goal of the research was to investigate whether or not aspirin prevented the formation of a clot around the catheter. As a matter of fact, the study confirmed that aspirin was indeed an antiplatelet agent, which we had known for a long time. It was finally 'proven' – but to achieve this, the right-hand chambers of the hearts of many 'consenting' patients had been cut into for no good reason.

The canons of die-hard mathematical methodology are now hammered into all medical students. We teach them that they must not believe what is not proven (and especially not believe the patient who is not reliable reproducible data!). A new discipline has emerged – 'critical article reading' – which now occupies a major place in the evaluation of students at the end of their medical studies. In substance, I find that critical reading is an excellent training that teaches students to take a different look at what is published. The problem is that it is being diverted from its original purpose to neutralise any personal reasoning by the physician.

The absurdity of purist reasoning, the 'blindness of the double-blind' that often prevails in medicine today, was perfectly pinned down by Smith and Pell in an article in the *British Medical Journal:* as a pastiche, they suggested listing the published objective data in order to determine to what extent a parachute fall is more effective than a free fall to reduce mortality or injuries if one jumps from an airplane. Owing to the fact that there some freefall survivors and some parachutists who died landing, or suffered 'side effects', such as a wide variety of injuries, the analysis found that there was a lack of objective data from which to draw any conclusions. The authors added that it was essential to find volunteers who had signed an informed consent form in order to set up a randomised study with a randomised intervention: in this case, jumping with a backpack equipped with a parachute against jumping with a backpack not containing a parachute (of course without the volunteers or the organisers knowing what each person's bag contained).

Medical research before randomised trials

I have often wondered how medicine made progress before the recent invention of randomised trials. In fact, disease management progressed through comparisons between medical schools. For a given complex illness, there would be a great boss who had 20 or 30 years of experience, who was challenged regularly by his younger assistants who had new ideas. In general, they did not have a ready-made recipe, but a decision-tree according to the different forms of the disease and the different features of the patients. There were often first-line treatments that did not work for everyone, then second- or third-line treatments. These strategies could include lifestyle changes (e.g. specific diets).

The big difference from the present time was that a medical professor at the head of a recognised school could publish his experience without any censorship. He simply, and almost always honestly, described his experience with his successes and failures. His colleagues from other schools could believe him or not, follow his example or not, but no one would have allowed themselves to prevent publication in a medical journal on the pretext that 'it is not possible' or that 'it is not formally and mathematically demonstrated'. Those who obtained the best results ended up pushing others to adopt their methods, for the greater good of the sick. There was no pressure to publish, unlike today when careers depend on publications ('publish or perish', as the Americans say). By practising in this way, there was no incentive to cheat; it had no allure. The situation has changed a lot because publication fraud is now becoming a colossal global problem to which research authorities have not found a solution. We catch only a minority of cheats. Anything that is not proven by mathematical criteria does not exist. The sick can die peacefully. In the early 1980s, one of my fellow residents, with whom I was on duty in the infectious disease intensive care ward in the former Claude-Bernard Hospital, wrote on the wall of the physicians' on-call room to paraphrase 'modern' medical practitice: 'A good post mortem is better than treatment without evidence'. It's cynical, but it is so true of some doctor's current medical reasoning.

Culture and medicine

Even if patients are now asked to give 'informed consent' to randomised trials, this sometimes causes more problems. Several times I have witnessed a different approach in patients of Anglo-Saxon culture from those of a Latin culture. In Latin culture, the doctor can be likened to the 'father' who holds knowledge and protects you. The conflict can be much greater with some African cultures. Thus, when the first active HIV drug, zidovudine (or AZT, Retrovir®), was available in France, it was initially only available in a randomised study in which half of the patients received a placebo. All the patients were informed about the randomisation but neither the patients nor the doctor knew what was inside the tablets. At the time, I was treating a young woman from the Ivory Coast, infected with HIV, who was studying at university level. She wanted to receive AZT.

I explained to her that, for a few months, while waiting for the results of the research, the only way to have a chance to get AZT was to enter the French-English clinical research trial called Concorde comparing the efficacy of AZT to that of a placebo. I gave her all the explanations. She looked at me astonished and coldly asked me this question: 'Are you really a doctor?' When I answered that as far as I knew I was, she added: 'You are a doctor and yet you don't even know what you are giving me to treat me, or if you are going to do me good or harm. It is not possible!' She got up and left. It was a culture shock for her. The doctor needs to be all-knowing.

Shortly afterwards, I was confronted with a serious problem by a patient of Tunisian origin, infected with HIV, at the AIDS (late symptomatic) stage. I had been treating him for almost a year and he had great confidence in me. One day, he developed a toxoplasma brain abscess as was common with this disease. He was hospitalised and unfortunately developed an allergy or side effects to any medication that could be offered to treat toxoplasmosis. It was possible to treat him with a new antibiotic that had already become commonplace in town and was frequently prescribed in private practice or in hospital for respiratory infections in adults or children. It was usually a well-tolerated medication with no annoying side effects. The only problem was that, in order to prescribe it for a prolonged period in toxoplasmosis, a temporary authorisation for use had to be requested from the Medicines Agency. It was a simple administrative procedure to obtain a very common drug, but informed consent had to be obtained from the patient.

Unfortunately, the fact that I was asking him to sign a piece of paper was interpreted by this patient as 'proof' that I considered him to be condemned to death in the short term since, in his head, a signature meant: 'I'm screwed, so they're experimenting on me and the doctor wants to absolve himself of his responsibility'. Overnight, this patient refused any help, any psychological support, any food, any medication and decided to die. Even though I and others talked to him for hours, he did not want to hear anything and did not trust us anymore. I have always thought, as his family confirmed to me, that asking for informed consent killed him. In his eyes I had changed his status from a human being to a guinea pig.

I will not even mention the many studies conducted in developing countries 'according to good clinical practice' on illiterate patients who put a cross in a box as signature without having understood anything.

At the beginning of my senior registrar period, Professor Marcel Francis Kahn, a great rheumatologist at the Bichat Hospital, often visited the Claude-Bernard Hospital to see patients hospitalised with various 'idiopathic' or 'autoimmune' diseases. He taught me a lot, and, with him, I observed the similarities between infectious diseases and idiopathic diseases. As I shared some of my thoughts with him, he encouraged me to read a remarkable book, *Medicine and Culture* by Lynn Payer. The author, an American journalist, studied the impact of different cultures on medical practices. She had in fact interviewed Kahn for her book. She had thereby compared medicine in the United States with several European countries, including France and Great Britain. This book is fascinating and is how I learned the origin of the placebo. For centuries, it has been well known that the French and English do not always had the same view of things. The French love to take tablets and when they think of a drug, it is first of all as a 'product that will do me good'. The English, on the other hand, think that the product may not work so well and may be the source of side effects, so they immediately wonder if it is really useful. Hence the need to evaluate against a placebo.

The worst thing for an English person, says the author – who deliberately relies on stereotypes to make this point – is to lose their self-control: in adversity it is necessary to maintain their composure and 'keep a stiff upper lip'. Nothing is worse, from this perspective, than to see someone get jittery and scream. Hence the large contribution of the English in the fields of pain relief and anaesthesia. The Americans, through their Anglo-Saxon culture, share the English point of view as to the need to prove the action of the drug. But, as observed by our investigator, the Americans differ from the English in that they spontaneously tend to consider themselves endowed with more strength than the other inhabitants of the planet, hence their subjective feeling of needing higher doses than the others, on a personal basis, even if it means exceeding the prescribed dose. If they are indeed not always stronger, they are often bigger than people in other countries; increasing the dose of a drug in cases of obesity can increase the risk of toxic effects. As a result, several drugs with a worldwide distribution have had to be withdrawn from the market because of side effects that only appeared in the United States. In fact, these accidents were related to patients deliberately overdosing, but that never prevented patients at fault from suing the drug manufacturers!

Similarly, American surgeons often cut wider than others. French surgeons are much more economical with their incisions. The French have made a much more artistic contribution to medicine. French doctors love to examine their patients from every angle. In comparison, English doctors, of a more prudish Puritan culture, do not touch their patients much and thus observe fewer signs.

As early as the nineteenth century, the French contributed greatly to the detailed clinical description of the signs and symptoms of diseases: they sometimes went so far as to speak as if describing a painting in an art gallery. Anglo-Saxons, more sceptical by nature, want incontravertible evidence, hence the acceptance of randomised trials. French doctors are very interested in the 'terrain' – that is, the individual as a whole, their family, personal history, way of life and underlying illnesses – and do not focus only on the disease in hand.

The difficulties of diagnosing and treating crypto-infections

Even when you believe that there is such a condition as chronic Lyme, the treatment is often not straightforward. Doctors who decide to risk diagnosing the disease are often satisfied to see their patients improve under antibiotic medication and they treat for a few months, but many fear exacerbations that they do not identify as such, but rather as 'side effects' of the drug and they then stop everything. Above all, my daring colleagues become disilluioned when they see most of the patients come back with a relapse. At that point, not knowing what to do and not wanting to hear about other treatment strategies that are not officially validated, they are desperate to get rid of the patient. If, by chance, another specialist makes a new diagnosis, this time officially recognised (depression, fibromyalgia, hypochondria, lupus, seronegative rheumatoid arthritis, reactive arthritis, tendonitis, or a well-known 'fashionable syndrome' of which 10 cases have been reported – see next), my colleagues are delighted to fall back on such and, especially, not to see the patient again. In fact, as I have already explained, to optimise the effectiveness of the treatment and avoid relapses, conventional antibiotics are not sufficient and other antimicrobial drugs, in particular antibiotics active on round persistent forms of *Borrelia*, antiparasitic agents and even some antifungals, play a major part in recovery.

'Macrophagic myofasciitis': a useful invention?

In the absence of efficient microbiological tools and in the face of patient confusion, hypotheses such as 'macrophagic myofasciitis' have been invented. 'Macrophagic myofasciitis' is a disease that has virtually only been reported in France by a particular group of doctors. Some physicians buried the infectious cause of this so-called 'new' disease to attack vaccines.

This diagnosis has been made in patients who had all the classic signs of fibromyalgia with some signs suggestive of autoimmune diseases such as lupus, rheumatoid arthritis and/or Hashimoto's thyroiditis. Several of the first patients described had stayed in tropical countries for a long time; some had a history of tuberculosis or sarcoidosis. Some had seen their muscle problems start after taking chloroquine or hydroxychloroquine. When the disease was first described in the *Lancet*, an infectious cause was mentioned, and patients improved with antibiotics. It was a 'new bacterial disease'; however it was not possible to isolate the responsible bacterium.

As this disease became fashionable among some hospital doctors, a larger number of patients with poorly identified muscle problems were diagnosed with it and treated with antibiotics. Next to the patients who improved on antibiotics, others, more numerous, worsened at the beginning of treatment, which does not surprise me when we know about the exacerbation reactions seen during the treatment of crypto-infections. The worsening of symptoms initially observed with the antimalarial drugs chloroquine or hydroxychloroquine, also probably corresponds to Jarisch-Herxheimer reactions, which are seen three times out of four during treatment of chronic Lyme disease.

Unfortunately, the 'invention' of 'macrophage myofasciitis' has done a great deal of harm to the cause of vaccinations in France and French-speaking countries, despite the fact that they apparently have nothing to do with this disease. For me, this entity is part of the crypto-infections group, and the few patients who had been diagnosed with it that I have treated have improved under prolonged antimicrobial treatment. One day when I was at a meeting on vaccinations with Professor Chérin, an ardent defender of this disease, he told me he had seen two of his patients whom I had treated for some time and who had improved well under antimicrobial treatments. He expressed his surprise. I then advised him to re-read his initial writings where he had evoked the infectious cause of the disease and the efficacy of antibiotics. Unfortunately, the promoters of this diagnosis who attribute it to vaccinations, do not suggest any solution and put the patients, who are really ill and suffering deeply, in a dead end without treatment.

Is aluminium responsible?

In the face of worsening symptoms in response to antimicrobial treatments, the infectious thesis to explain 'macrophagic myofasciitis' was abandoned very quickly – far too quickly. The theory that aluminium, commonly used as an 'adjuvant' (immune stimulus) in vaccinations was responsible, advanced by an anatomo-pathologist, was not established either. It looks for an inflammatory reaction around traces of aluminium remaining in the injection zone of vaccines (usually the deltoid muscle). The problem is that almost the entire population has received many vaccines, representing billions of people worldwide. Thus, many people in the world have traces of aluminium in their deltoid muscle. If aluminium had been found in the diseased muscles, one might have believed this hypothesis, but in fact not the slightest trace of aluminium has been found in these muscles. The causal link of aluminium to this rare disease, described almost exclusively in France, could never be shown.

Aluminium is not a heavy metal but, on the contrary, a particularly light metal. Unlike heavy metals, aluminium, which represents 8 to 9% of the earth's crust, has been present everywhere in the natural environment since time immemorial. It is the third most common element on earth after oxygen and silicon. It is the most abundant metal in nature. The earth's crust is full of aluminium. It is everywhere, in the soil, in water, in plants. There is much more aluminium than there is iron or coal. Many healthy vegetables contain significant amounts of aluminium. This has nothing to do with the modern world, industrial pollution, the invention of aluminium pots and pans, beer or soda cans, or tin foil for baking. It is important to emphasise this when reading on 'organic' websites that cooking fish in foil can cause paralysis! The most organic food in the world contains aluminium – for example, tea, which is one of the most widely consumed products and contains the highest levels (over 2%). Every day we eat between 5 and 12 milligrammes of aluminium per kilogramme of food.

Thus, the traces of aluminium present in many vaccines do not represent much compared with all the aluminium that we ingest every day. It is true that only a tiny part is absorbed by the digestive tract, but we consume it every day for decades.

The small amount absorbed each day is quickly eliminated in our urine. In the brains of people who have died at a very old age, traces of aluminium are very often found, but this seems logical, given the permanent exposure in the environment. This has nothing to do with the neurological toxicity of aluminium which does exist at very high doses and which was described at the beginning of artificial kidney haemodialysis when patients could have huge aluminium overdoses. Some then claimed that aluminium was the cause of Alzheimer's disease. However, the infectious cause of Alzheimer's is now established.

There are no simple answers

The National Reference Centre (NRC) for Borreliosis at the Pasteur Institute and then at Strasbourg have always obeyed IDSA, standing to attention at whatever they recommend, and no French microbiologist has taken an interest in this subject. For example, as I mentioned earlier, Professor Didier Raoult, a well-known specialist in tick-borne infections, has never accepted the existence of chronic Lyme. It is a pity because this microbiologist is very active and full of ideas, he is surrounded by many quality researchers and has considerable resources for his laboratory. As I admired his dynamism and had a very friendly relationship with him, I tried to raise his awareness by going to Marseille with my collaborator Jérôme Salomon who, since the beginning, has tried to help me get some sound care for patients. Didier Raoult has, however, stuck with the view: one germ for one pathology, 'Christian, define a syndrome for me with very specific criteria, Garches' syndrome', he said with a smile. 'Your criteria should not overlap with another disease. Then, when your objective criteria are well defined, let me know and I'll help you find the bacteria responsible for Garches' syndrome'.

I answered that for me, the patients presented far too diverse a clinical picture and that I no longer believed in the simplistic theory: one germ, one pathology. To me, these complex situations are linked to a mingling of factors with possible simultaneous involvement of several microbes. Didier concluded that my patients complained of signs that were too varied and non-specific and that he could do nothing about them. So, I left well alone.

In 2020, I met Didier to speak about the Covid-19 crisis. He beautifully confirmed the activity of hydroxychloroquine against Covid-19, already demonstrated by Chinese experts, and showed its synergistic activity when combined with azithromycin. Thus, an anti-parasitic drug and an antibiotic have antiviral properties against the new coronavirus SARS-CoV-2. He gave me a copy of the book that he had just published about epidemics (*Epidémies: vrais dangers et fausses alertes*) and I was glad to read in it that he no longer believed in the theory of one germ, one pathology. He also seemed convinced that patients suffering from polymorphic signs and symptoms are not psychiatric cases but their problems have an organic cause. He also recognised that *Rickettsiae* may persist.

Infectious diseases versus clinical microbiology

The simplistic vision of trying to find a single germ for a pathology illustrates the limits of medical microbiology. Previously, physicians who had received solid clinical training at the bedside could also pursue their careers in microbiology laboratories while continuing their clinical activity. That was quite possible even 25 years ago. Given the modern constraints of the professions on both sides, the laboratory profession, which has become highly specialised, and the profession at patients' bedsides, which requires the constant enrichment of one's experience and diagnostic 'flair', it becomes impossible to do both properly. It is not enough to read the antibiotic sensitivity test of a bacterium isolated from a patient to treat him or her. Moreover, the vast majority of microbiologists today are no longer doctors but pharmacists, who do not have the right to practise medicine. That is why the 'infectious diseases' specialty, which is a clinical discipline, is now recognised in most countries, though not evident in those where infectious diseases were to be eradicated (in the minds of decision-makers).

I was involved for several years, with Daniel Christmann from Strasbourg, within the European Union of Medical Specialists (UEMS), in the defence and promotion of the specialty 'infectious diseases' in all countries of the European Union. It was a great joy for Daniel and me that we helped our German colleagues, especially Professor Winfried Kern, in the recognition of the discipline in their country a few years ago. Only two countries in Europe still do not recognise the speciality: Belgium and Spain. In France, I fought with the help of colleagues so that infectious and tropical diseases, which had been a complementary sub-specialty, finally became a full specialty in 2015.

It is not surprising to note that countries where so-called 'clinical' microbiology remains predominant over infectious diseases, such as Great Britain and the Nordic countries, are the countries where the situation of patients suffering from chronic Lyme disease is most critical. The current biological tests being unreliable, results are often negative. Thus, physicians who are mainly lab doctors only consider proven biological data, and don't recognise any organic disease if tests are negative. The recently formed European Society for Clinical Microbiology and Infectious Diseases (ESCMID) is dominated by 'clinical microbiologists' which explains their lack of understanding of chronic Lyme disease, which at present should be diagnosed clinically (that is, on the basis of symptoms, not blood tests). This Society recently created a working group on borreliosis (ESGBOR), which replaced EUCALB (European Union Concerted Action on Lyme Borreliosis) which disappeared in 2017. ESGBOR, against scientific evidence, continues to follow the now obsolete IDSA guidelines.

Chapter 11

Hope

Raising awareness

Lyme disease has not interested scientists for decades, let alone journalists. Talking about Lyme was a guaranteed flop. I also discovered over the years that the editors of medical journals had been well 'briefed' by 'experts' on the IDSA dogma: 'Lyme is a rare disease that is diagnosed and treated without problems and without relapse; 'chronic Lyme' is the fabrication of a few hypochondriacs and charlatan doctors'. Chronic Lyme was on the list of subjects to avoid at all costs.

A few years ago, the journalists of a famous television show devoted to quality reporting interviewed me at length and discovered with great interest the 'world of chronic Lyme'. They had an ambitious project consisting of interviews with experts in France and abroad as well as patients. The report was never shot. 'Experts' contacted by the journalists to be interviewed had immediately moved heaven and earth to block the shooting at the highest level of the channel. I discovered that Lyme censorship was being exercised not only by medical journals, but also on mainstream media. I have witnessed this type of censorship on several occasions. Fortunately, reality is stronger than censorship, which is becoming fractured and cracking open. We can finally talk about Lyme in the newspapers and on television.

Raising political awareness

As I mentioned earlier, local regional politicians have been aware of the Lyme disease problem for years in diverse regions of the country. In their constituencies, there are many farmers, hunters, tourists and sports people engaged in outdoor activities. They have seen the abandonment of their sick citizens by doctors. I do not want to accuse local doctors of bad practice, as for the most part they do not know about this disease. When they encounter a case (usually it is the patient or family member who has made the diagnosis), they follow official recommendations. Those doctors who are convinced that these recommendations are totally inadequate do not dare to offer different treatments, or they do so clandestinely. Several doctors are currently subject to disciplinary proceedings for not following the recommendations.

As outlined in Chapter 6, the political turnaround began in several states in the United States (Virginia in January 2013, Vermont in March 2014, then New York State in January 2015), where laws were passed recognising chronic Lyme. In the summer of 2016, 15 American states passed Lyme legislation. This is a major political recognition, and in some states, legislation now requires that patients are informed that diagnostic antibody tests are not reliable. These laws call for some research funding to develop new tests and treatment strategies and an end to the persecution of 'crypto-infectiologists', the courageous doctors who care for patients with chronic Lyme disease and co-infections. Insurance companies are compelled to reimburse antimicrobial treatments beyond three weeks in these states. At the federal level, a law was passed unanimously in the House of Representatives in September 2014 and the US Federal law was voted in December 2016. A Lyme law was passed in Canada in December 2014 unanimously by the Canadian Senate.

In France, however, when the High Council of Public Health published a damning report on the current situation, although 70 deputies supported a vote on a law for Lyme disease, the Secretary of State for Handicap, Ségolène Neuville (an infectious disease doctor), told the National Assembly, with the support of the Minister for Health, Marisol Touraine, that there was no problem with Lyme in France, and the deputies of the Socialist majority party were instructed to block the bill. A Socialist MP wrote to me, confused, to say that he had been sorry to be forced to follow his party's voting instructions, but that he strongly encouraged me to keep going with my legitimate fight. Most curiously, since this parliamentary debate, eminent political figures have contacted me regularly to ask me to see people they know who suffer from chronic Lyme disease. Strange for an imaginary disease!

The only consolation after this parliamentary debacle is that, in return, the Minister for Health announced that she would help support research. Again, strange for a disease that does not exist! Given the impossibility of obtaining public funding for research, whether in France or in other countries, particularly in the United States, the announcement by the French Minister for Health that she would ensure funding in this area was an excellent piece of news for patients. I welcomed this progress and the apparent increase in awareness of this problem by the Minister's office and the General Directorate for Health. Strong political impetus is needed to come to the rescue of the sick. Unfortunately in 2018, nothing good happened. Funding for research remained very low and actions were blocked by learned societies. I'll go into more details in the last chapter.

In September 2015, thanks to the energetic work of some dynamic Belgian researchers, Valérie Obsomer, entomologist, and Liesbeth Borgermans, doctor in medical sciences and professor in chronic care in the Department of Family Medicine at the Université Libre de Bruxelles, Richard Horowitz and I were invited to a hearing before the Committee on Public Health, the Environment and the Renewal of Society of the Belgian House of Representatives. Liesbeth and Valerie asked me to join them with two other colleagues (Ran Balicer from Ben Gurion University of Negev in Israel and Ozren Polacek from the University of Split in Croatia, and who was also working in a global health research centre at Edinburgh University in Scotland) to write an editorial for the prestigious *British Medical Journal* (BMJ). The title of the article was: *'Lyme disease: time for a new approach?'*[1] This publication, accepted by the journal, gave us great pleasure, because it is exceptional for experts 'from the opposition to established dogma' to succeed in publishing in such a widely read journal, the *BMJ* being, in 2015, ranked fifth in the world among general medical journals.

In February 2016, a petition launched by a courageous patient from Luxembourg, Tania Silva, mother of two children, achieved unexpected success. Given the enormous number of signatories, the Chamber of Deputies of Luxembourg received the petition representatives, who had asked me to accompany them. The Minister for Health and the Minister for Social Security of Luxembourg were present and were able to listen to our arguments. I then learned with astonishment that a Lyme diagnosis was almost never made in Luxembourg and that there had been officially three cases during the previous year and zero cases two years before. Strange in a country where ticks in the surrounding territories are hyper-contaminated. On a political level, I appreciated that a small country had a very democratic way of functioning, with the possibility of direct contact between complainants and ministers or the President of the Chamber of Deputies.

In Canada, after the Lyme Act was passed, new recommendations were developed with the help of 'crypto-infectiologists'. Unfortunately, the Canadian recommendations remained rather similar to the IDSA guidelines.

In the United States, the official website that hosts national recommendations for health professionals and insurance companies, the National Guidelines Clearinghouse (NGC), in 2017, removed the obsolete recommendations from the IDSA expert group, not validated by the Institute of Medicine, and then displayed only those from ILADS, a learned society that for years had been accused of advocating 'anti-science' (see page 105). It is a fitting reversal of roles, and American patients could rejoice. However, for budgetary reasons, the NGC was suppressed.

Paradoxically, the anti-chronic Lyme lobby in Europe has become more entrenched. One example is the tendentious use of a report from the European Centre for Disease Prevention and Control (ECDC), published in April 2016. This report stressed the many problems arising from blood serum antibody testing, and the fact that it was not calibrated on well defined groups of patients or healthy 'control' individuals. Thus they emphasised the need to compare its results with the clinical signs of patients and concluded that the indications they provided should be used with caution pending more solid data. Yet, this report has been used by 'experts', notably in France, to say that the ECDC 'has demonstrated' that blood testing is perfect. In fact, these 'experts' only looked at the annexes to the report, where data from the test manufacturers suggested excellent test sensitivity – data criticised in the report.

The fact that politicians in many countries are increasingly pushing for recognition of Lyme disease should make them aware of the need to fund research and facilitate the establishment of independent international working groups. Thus, scientists could take control of the situation again. Reliable tests are essential to study many unclear syndromes that can simulate other diseases. There is an urgent need to foster basic and clinical research as that would be the most cost-effective way to ensure that patients are diagnosed, and the best therapeutic strategies are developed.

In recent years, there has been a growing annual event in many countries, the World-Wide Lyme Protest (WWLP), a protest against global Lyme borreliosis denial.

The swansong of the anti-Lyme IDSA clique?

Attacked from all sides and no longer having the institutional support of the American authorities, the IDSA Lyme expert group intensified its activities to justify itself in the eyes of history. An example of this can be seen in a study published in 2016 by Berende in the *New England Journal of Medicine,* with an editorial by Michael Melia and Paul Auwaerter.[152] The title of the editorial, 'Time for a different approach to Lyme disease and long-term symptoms', seemed all the more promising as it largely followed the formula chosen by Liesbeth Borgermans, myself and other collaborators for our own editorial published in December 2015 in the *British Medical Journal* that I have already mentioned. There is now indeed a global consensus on a multifactorial approach to the disease and associated diseases due to co-infections by microbes other than *Borrelia burgdorferi.* The problem for patients is that the IDSA authors only copied the title. I would have forgiven them for plagiarising the whole article and would even, to tell you the truth, have been grateful!

Unfortunately, the study by Berende and his collaborators did not provide any answers to all the questions raised by recent scientific publications which proved the persistence of *Borrelia,* even after a few months of antibiotic treatment, and the capacity of the bacterium to take various forms to better persist in the cells and tissues of its 'host', whether animal or human, as some authors have shown.[77, 154, 173] After two weeks of an injectable antibiotic, ceftriaxone, patients were randomly allocated between three groups. Over the next three months, one group would receive placebo, the second group an oral antibiotic, doxycycline, and the third group the combination of an oral antibiotic, clarithromycin and hydroxychloroquine (Plaquenil®), a potent antimicrobial as described above. These two anti-infective treatment strategies are adapted for the treatment of Lyme disease.

Why did they stop the treatment and the evaluation of the patients at three months? We know that at this time point, in the experience of all physicians caring for chronic Lyme, we are still in a phase where exacerbations of signs and symptoms triggered by treatments (the Jarisch-Herxheimer reaction or 'herx') remain present in a significant proportion of patients, who will improve significantly or even recover a few weeks or months later.

Moreover, there was nothing in the study methods used by the IDSA authors to differentiate exacerbations of the disease from the true side effects of antimicrobial drugs. Only the extension of treatment beyond three months has shown that these so-called 'side effects' eventually disappear while the same treatment is continued.

The study did not take into account the natural cyclical evolution of the disease, which is very frequent, so that at three months, independently of treatment, some patients will be in a phase of exacerbation and others in a phase of regression of their symptoms. Experience has shown that these oscillations usually end up, under prolonged treatment, being less strong and less frequent over time, and eventually, in the best cases, disappear after a few months. The study seemed to start well with an analysis of the signs and symptoms from which the patients suffered at baseline, before starting treatments. So far, so good, but once patients were randomly assigned to one of the three groups, their signs and symptoms were no longer monitored or analysed at all. The authors were satisfied with an overall quality of life score, the SF36, which established an average of the general state felt by the patients without any detail on their different categories of signs and symptoms. These may be general signs (fatigue, fever, sweating, weight variations) or signs affecting different body systems: skin, joints, muscles, bone, heart, neurological, etc. All these signs absolutely cannot be evaluated individually by the SF36 score.

Thus, for physicians who are perfectly familiar with the management of chronic Lyme, this method of evaluation can show nothing useful at three months. Patients in the placebo group, after perhaps a small initial improvement due to the two weeks of ceftriaxone, remained fairly stable or resumed the natural oscillations of their clinical signs. Patients in groups receiving a real antimicrobial treatment would normally be divided into three subgroups, but this was absolutely not studied in the IDSA work: those who showed good improvement, those who were in a worse state than before the start of treatment (because of exacerbations) and those in whom certain categories of signs had improved while others were in a phase of aggravation. For example, at three months, a patient might notice a marked improvement in joint pain and a virtual disappearance of heart problems, while their headaches and intellectual fog might be even worse than before treatment. Overall, the patient would say they were not feeling well, and their SF36 score would be bad but they might have recovered three months later.

The authors of this study were well aware that the methodology they used was unable to show a difference between the groups at three months. They knew this because they copied the methodology already used 15 years ago by Klempner and his collaborators. This earlier study, which included only two groups (antibiotic versus placebo), published in 2001, as if by chance, in the same journal, the *New England Journal of Medicine*, had shown no difference between the groups. From this point of view, it was foreseeable that Berende's new study, because of the way it had been designed, would contribute nothing new.

On top of that, it was interesting to note that a proportion of the patients included in the study had had a negative Lyme antibody test. This is not shocking in itself, and one might even rejoice, but it is incomprehensible from experts who say that Lyme antibody tests are perfect. Once more, spot the mistake.

While at the American and international level it is required more and more that patient-support associations be consulted on the recommendations that affect them, whatever the disease, it is astonishing to note that patients suffering from chronic Lyme disease did not have a say in the design of the study and that the opinion of many Lyme doctors was not sought for the methodology. These numerous Lyme doctors take care of patients worldwide and they have cured hundreds of thousands of patients suffering from persistent disabling signs and symptoms. Many published studies have shown the benefit of prolonged antibiotic treatment, with an enhanced effect by adding hydroxychloroquine.[2, 18, 70, 71] Randomised studies comparing an antibiotic with a placebo have shown efficacy by measuring specific signs and not a vague quality of life score.[80, 123] In Fallon's study, improvements in cognitive impairment were measured with objective tests and correlated with changes in brain blood flow measured by SPECT scan (single-photon emission tomography).

We can therefore conclude that Berende and colleagues' study was deliberately designed to show nothing. Thus, 15 years after Klempner's study, this was its only lazy reply. The same old story. I thought, and hoped that this lamentable article would prove to be the 'swan song' of the IDSA Lyme clique, but in fact IDSA changed nothing and continues to influence the medical world.

Current treatment recommendations

As with tuberculosis and other persistent infections with a prolonged evolution, it is clear that two phases of treatment are necessary. During the first, corresponding to the induction therapy, antibiotics classically recommended for being active on bacteria in their growth phase, with rapid multiplication, can be used. When the infection has calmed down and the symptoms have decreased, it is essential to change the rationale and move on to a second phase, corresponding to maintenance therapy (this is the 'maintenance phase' I have mentioned earlier), by favouring antibiotics or other antimicrobials active against persistent bacteria in their latent phase. These 'sleeping' bacteria have a slowed metabolism or are in the 'round' form I described earlier and thus escape the action of antibiotics. Clinical research is needed to evaluate these maintenance treatment strategies.

Other factors that may affect the disease

Great heat, or on the contrary, great cold, can have a beneficial effect in some patients. This does not surprise me because thermal shocks were used before the era of antibiotics to treat tertiary syphilis, based on the work of the neuropsychiatrist Julius Wagner-Jaurreg. Wagner-Jaurreg has been widely criticised for using electric shock therapy on patients in barbaric conditions. Soldiers who had suffered emotional trauma linked to the war preferred to return to the front-line, and the hell of the trenches, rather than to remain in psychiatry in the hands of this doctor, although fellow-psychiatrist, Freud, did defend his work. But apart from his work with electric shocks, Wagner-Jaurreg's theories on thermal shock were well established scientifically. Syphilis, like Lyme, is caused by a temperature-sensitive spirochete.

Some prefer cryotherapy to heat, where the body is immersed at –150°C for less than three minutes. (Interestingly, this is current practice for intensively trained sports people, cyclists among others.)

In some cases, a change of diet can improve the clinical condition of patients over the long term, in particular reducing the intake of gluten, non-fermented dairy products, sugar and red meat. This is in line with current studies of the composition of the intestinal flora (the so-called 'microbiota'), which seems to modulate the evolution of certain chronic diseases.

There are several teams around the world working on the modification of the microbiota and the evolution of various chronic diseases. Experiments in faecal transplantation have been carried out, where a faecal sample from a healthy donor is inoculated into the sick recipient, often through a nasogastric tube. Recently, there was a publication from a research team that administered intestinal worms not dangerous for humans to patients with an autoimmune disease. This implantation of parasites has had a beneficial effect on chronic disease in some recipients. RM Maizels published a review about the interactions between intestinal worms, allergy and auto-immune diseases.[140a]

Poisoning from heavy metals such as lead and mercury (not aluminium, which, as explained in the previous chapter, is a naturally light metal and is omnipresent in food), in particular from dental fillings, could play a part in some cases, but this remains difficult to evaluate in France because practice and research on the topic are prohibited. In France, this type of investigation is done only clandestinely. However, research into the effect of heavy metals used in dental work is carried out openly elsewhere, notably in Germany, Switzerland, Spain and the United States. The efficiency of removing these metals (chelations) varies. I have seen patients spend a lot of money without any results and, conversely, I have seen some dramatic improvements in clinical condition after amalgam removal and chelation.

French doctors no longer dare to get involved in this field; one with the greatest experience, an epidemiologist, Jean-Jacques Melet, committed suicide in 2005 after he was persecuted by the health authorities. Of course, we must remain cautious in this area and put things into perspective, because billions of people in the world have dental amalgams, and overall life expectancy around the world is increasing. Since the problem only affects certain individuals, genetic susceptibility to heavy metals should not be excluded. This area deserves to be taken out of the shadows and subjected to serious evaluation.

With the development of bacterial resistance to antibiotics, a movement is emerging among doctors and scientists in several countries to revive research on bacteriophages. Bacteriophages are small viruses capable of attacking bacteria and, during the first half of the twentieth century, they were successfully used to treat various serious infections. This method of treatment, called phage therapy, almost disappeared in industrialised countries after the appearance of antibiotics. Only countries of the former Soviet Union and Eastern Europe that were under Soviet influence retained some of the tradition of phage therapy. An English team is developing an anti-*Borrelia burgdorferi* bacteriophage, but further research is needed to allow bacteriophages to enter human cells where *Borreliae* are hidden. The search for bacteriophages, specific for *Borreliae* in the blood, is being developed as a diagnostic test. As bacteriophages living on *Borreliae* are much more numerous than their bacterial partners, they are easier to isolate, and their presence is the proof that the bacteria are present.

Evidence-based medicine: for better or for worse

I have observed clear improvements or cures of chronic Lyme disease and also of other varied diseases due to my antimicrobial treatments. Despite incomprehension from my French colleagues, I have been comforted by later meeting doctors from other countries who have had the same experience as myself, and who also could not publish their results. So, I was not the only crazy person.

In the world, there are millions of patients and thousands of 'crypto-infectiologists' who treat them daily and cure a large number of them. Yet these doctors are not recognised. The system refuses to see that there are people who are suffering and people who know how to treat them.

As outlined in the previous chapter, the whole research system is organised around the simplistic concept of one cause, one disease. Yet many patients do not fit this picture. By prioritising only objective, scientifically measurable criteria, the personal criteria of the physician are marginalised.

Freedom of expression hardly exists any more in the modern standardised system of scientific publication, where everything has to be perfectly proven before discussion can take place. This was not the case in the days of our former bosses who were free to publish their experience in medical journals, even when it was atypical. Certainly, medicine is a science, which must be as accurate as possible, but not everything is completely demonstrable in medicine with current tools. Fortunately, medicine is also an art, but we tend to forget this.

In his book *La Médecine Expérimentale (Experimental Medicine),* Claude Bernard described a scientific methodology based on experimental evidence used in the nineteenth century. Claude Bernard, who absolutely wanted this evidence, often defended the 'spontaneous generation' of certain diseases before it was possible to 'prove' the existence of the responsible microbes. Despite his 'Doubting Thomas' way of thinking – 'I only believe what I can see' – I have a lot of respect for Claude Bernard, thanks to his innovative thinking, the former infectious diseases hospital in Paris bore his name. He laid the foundations for medical experimentation. More recently, the need for evidence has led to the concept of 'evidence-based medicine'.

When I became interested in evidence-based medicine, I was surprised to discover that one of the Canadian promoters of this approach, David Sackett, urged experts to remember that evidence-based medicine was more than just following raw data from the medical literature, including randomised studies and in particular meta-analyses (rigorous scientific analyses of a set of publications on the same subject in an attempt to synthesise them). Evidence-based medicine was in fact a combination of each physician's individual clinical experience and the evidence provided by available external sources (basic scientific data, clinically relevant research results). Often, these available data are incomplete, may be of poor quality and do not always capture the whole problem. Individual clinical experience, according to Sackett, means the competence and individual judgement of the clinician acquired over time through practice with patients. The third ingredient of evidence-based medicine was patient choice. Sackett concluded that evidence-based medicine could in no way be an unthinking follow up of ready-made recipes in the form of recommendations or guidelines. He insisted that the patient's choice should never be forgotten. He also predicted that the last two ingredients would likely be forgotten over time. This doctor was a prophet!

Needless to say, the third ingredient of evidence-based medicine is currently ignored by most physicians. The experienced patient is seen by many doctors as a troublemaker. Doctors prefer to look at scans and laboratory results rather than to listen to the patient's complaints or wishes. The better informed a patient is, and the more s/he knows the medical publications concerning his/her disease, the faster s/he is 'reframed' by the doctor. Questions or requests for clarification are often perceived by the doctor as inappropriate, especially if the patient expresses the slightest objection. This phenomenon has increased with the internet because, in some cases, and I see it every day, smart patients know much more than the doctor. Such patients are often disposed of by referral to a psychiatrist or other specialist.

The second ingredient of evidence-based medicine is, in addition to the third, totally ignored by health authorities.

Medical Councils, health insurers and some courts now look only at the scientific literature, 'expert' recommendations and consensus conferences. It is not medicine anymore! To return to Lyme disease, it should be recalled, once again, that a scientific publication published in a major American medical journal has shown that most of the IDSA recommendations that have had the force of law in the world of Lyme disease and that were included in the 2006 French Consensus Conference are not in any way based on evidence but on the opinion of a few American experts.

Non-randomised studies should be published

When a study does not include a randomised trial, it is not even read, as it is not seen as science and does not lead to a 'reliable' conclusion. However, this consensus is not always followed. As an astonishing example, the world medical community has accepted the standards of treatment for chronic Q fever (caused by *Coxiella burnetii* infection) based on open studies with a relatively low number of patients, without any randomised trial. Why is it that for this chronic infection, specialists are happy to give 18 months of antibiotic treatment 'without proof', instead of abandoning the patients to their fate, according to their cherished international standards of evaluation?

I'm very happy that patients with chronic Q fever have access to an 18-month course of a combination of doxycycline and hydroxychloroquine, but, despite this combination often being very successful for treating chronic Lyme disease, it is not 'authorised'. Why? Several open studies of chronic Lyme cases show the benefits of prolonged tetracycline therapy (doxycycline is a tetracycline antibiotic) and of combining an antibiotic with hydroxychloroquine. The reason this treatment is not authorised for Lyme disease is the lack of a good randomised study of sufficient duration to prove its effectiveness. The example of these two chronic bacterial infections shows that there are – yet again – double standards being applied, according to some opinion leaders active in the field.

There are other examples of this double standard, including Whipple's disease (mentioned earlier – page 223), which is a whole-body disease caused by the bacterium *Tropheryma whipplei*. The main signs are arthritis, weight loss, abdominal pain and diarrhoea. The recommended antibiotic treatment consists of several weeks of penicillin or ceftriaxone intravenously, followed by at least one year of cotrimoxazole (sulphonamide) or a combination of doxycycline and hydroxychloroquine. In addition, relapses after treatment have been described in some patients and, in these cases, further treatment is accepted by the medical community, including even lifelong antibiotic treatment.

Sciatica of the lumbar spine is another example of probable bacterial involvement in a disease. A study of volunteer sciatica patients comparing an antibiotic treatment, doxycycline, with a placebo demonstrated the efficacy of this antibiotic in the treatment of sciatica. Surgical sampling of vertebral discs obtained from patients before treatment showed the presence of a bacterium, usually causing acne, *Propionibacterium acnes.* As this bacterium is often found on healthy skin, one might wonder if the samples had been contaminated, which is always possible. The disturbing fact is that it was found on different samples. Whatever the microbe(s) involved, the important fact is the demonstration of the efficacy of antibiotic treatment. It seems to me that it is a priority to repeat similar studies to confirm the results. The rheumatologists I know who have read the study have quickly put it in a drawer and do not want to hear about antibiotic treatment for sciatica or low back pain generally.

Medical innovation does not depend on randomised trials

One example of the excessive use of randomised trials is HIV-AIDS research, which is in the hands of the pharmaceutical industry. Dr Jacques Leibowitch, who continued to work in Garches despite having officially retired, and who died in 2020, was a genius who was always ahead in the field of HIV. As Luc Montagnier, discoverer of HIV and Nobel Prize winner, confirmed to me, Leibowitch contributed to the discovery of HIV by putting researchers on the trail of a retrovirus that could be the root of AIDS. He saw before anyone else the imperfection of the blood test used at the beginning. He went against the entire medical establishment to denounce the abuse of placebo and 'control groups' receiving a single drug with the certainty of rapidly selecting resistant HIV viruses. Fundamentalist 'methodologists' had already taken over humanist physicians in the field of research, much to the delight of drug manufacturers.

When I arrived at Garches in 1994, all HIV patients treated by Leibowitch had regular blood viral load measurements to monitor the effectiveness of antiretroviral therapy in real time. Helped by Dominique Mathez, he used this technique, then unique in the world, routinely. This was not known because Leibowitch, always in the heat of the moment, did not like to publish the results of his research. At Garches, he carried out the world's first treatment protocol using a combination of three antiretroviral drugs, the famous triple therapies. This was the trial he called Stalingrad because it was the turning point in his war on HIV.

When, a few years later, he told me about his successful antiretroviral drug reduction trials, the ICCARRE strategy for 'intermittent and short, antiretrovirals remain effective,' I was enthusiastic and immediately decided to help him with this endeavour. All his prescriptions were, of course. outside official medicine authorisation. Jacques Leibowitch and I were aggressively accused by some of my infectious disease colleagues of being insane in supporting a dangerous treatment. I convinced Jacques to publish his results, which we did with two articles in a prestigious international immunology journal, the *FASEB Journal*.[145a]

This strategy, which greatly reduced the quantity of drugs absorbed, was not viewed very favourably by pharmaceutical companies yet it was further validated in an official trial promoted by the National Agency for AIDS Research (ANRS), published in 2017 in the *Journal of Antimicrobial Chemotherapy*.[68a] This success encouraged us to remain open-minded and not to blindly follow the mainstream or some lobbies. Now this innovative strategy, considered as real progress in the management of HIV infection by the medical community, has been further evaluated in a double-blind randomised study.

Unfortunately, it is difficult to replicate this approach when studying Lyme disease. Due to the official position on Lyme disease and the threat of persecution by health authorities, there is a glaring lack of trained 'crypto-infectiologists'. Doctors are not rushing forward to volunteer. However, more and more doctors are interested, especially after seeing affected patients in their clinics. Many would like to take care of these patients, but they are afraid, and I can understand why. Although I knew some university hospital colleagues who confessed to me in private that they were 'doing a bit of chronic Lyme' in secret, no academic wanted to follow in my footsteps.

Yet I know from some colleagues and patients that some doctors who shout loudly and clearly in public that chronic Lyme does not exist sneak around treating patients with several months of antibiotics. They do not want anyone to know; it would damage their image. I am not here to 'expose' them. Outside Garches, no head of department, academic or otherwise, dares to make a commitment. The only exception in France is Dr Raouf Ghozzi, who was head of the internal medicine department at the Lannemezan Hospital Centre in the Hautes-Pyrénées.

Fortunately, there are many general practitioners who courageously accept the care of patients at their peril. I pay them an admiring and sincere tribute because they now practise in fear. It is of the utmost urgency to stop their persecution.

Of course, these treatments, if they are to remain flexible and open, must be supervised by a serious follow-up network with clinical reference centres, so that 'crypto-infectiology' does not fall into the hands of opportunistic charlatans who would like to make money on the backs of patients in distress.

Improving the training of doctors and the organisation of care

As soon as the authorities have given the necessary instructions to stop the witch-hunt and restore reimbursements for treatment, many hospital and private doctors will volunteer to help with the care of patients in pain. Unfortunately, many of these doctors will be lost sailing in unknown waters; they will not be able to see that the patient consulting them really has seronegative chronic Lyme, or another crypto-infection. Even if they do extend the antibiotic treatment, they will be destabilised by initial worseing of symptoms and relapses. The disease is chronic, usually life-long, and requires learning to become familiar with all the ingredients of management. Indeed, today, in the absence of steering tools, navigation is done 'on sight' with strategies developed 'à la carte'. As no two patients ever respond in the same way, probably because of the multiplicity of factors involved, it is necessary to constantly adapt according to the response to each treatment line and also according to the overall evolution of symptoms. The 'crypto-infectiologists' will have to set up training courses for their colleagues.

It will take years for most physicians to accept a challenge to their usual practices. The most effective strategy would be to open specialised units or health centres where volunteer and motivated physicians could be recruited. To advance research, these centres should work in networks to share medical data and protocols. The establishment of a national cohort of patients, with the support of the authorities, seems to be a priority. As detailed further on, such centres were created in France in 2019 by the Ministry of Health, but under the authority of infectious disease professors who did not believe in chronic Lyme disease and followed the IDSA way of thinking. It was a shock and considered a betrayal by Lyme patients and the wider Lyme community.

This management of crypto-infections will have to give a large place to preventive medicine, by integrating in particular new knowledge on diets and the composition of the intestinal flora (microbiota), on the links with nature and in particular knowledge of arthropod vectors, such as ticks, and certain forms of natural medicine such as phytotherapy.

Mobilising the pharmaceutical industry

For pharmaceutical companies, chronic diseases are a good investment because the duration of treatment is unlimited. Manufacturers who have a commercial commitment to their shareholders will not spontaneously favour research when it tends to lighten treatments, revalidate old, cheap drugs or, 'worse', cure these chronic diseases. However, it must be understood that the industry is an absolutely essential partner in advancing research. It is thanks to the pharmaceutical industry that considerable medical progress has been made. Only the industry has the capital and the technical means to invent and make available new diagnostic tests or new treatments, but, admittedly, the economic constraints are tremendous.

Developing new drugs is becoming more and more expensive and many products do not complete their development and are never marketed. This is often the case when an unexpected rare side effect is discovered at the end of the process, just at the time of commercialisation. Failure to develop a product can jeopardise the company's survival. The role of public research agencies and researchers themselves is to try to channel industrial research and to convince them that new strategies can also allow a return on investment. Medical ethics must play a major part here because ethical values often struggle against capitalist constraints.

For Lyme disease, manufacturers are not investing because they are told that it is a rare disease that gets cured in three weeks with old antibiotics that cost a few pounds. Moreover, they have seen the fierce global controversy that is scaring away investors. When the industry realises that crypto-infections affect millions and more likely billions of people around the world, that multiple microbes are involved, and that a range of diagnostic tests must be developed, the outlook on Lyme disease and related conditions will change overnight. When they understand that these are real chronic infections, difficult, even sometines impossible, to cure completely, they will invest in research into new antibacterial, antiparasitic, antifungal and even antiviral drugs. A new research field is opening up with the development of a whole range of maintenance treatments to keep symptoms at bay. Firms will get real returns on their investment. Since 2018 we can see that some manufacturers have been discovering this huge field and some have started investing in research. That is really good news.

Changing paradigms in research

It is necessary to prioritise the development of new diagnostic methods. These new techniques, sometimes already used in veterinary medicine, should be applied to humans. Other determinants, such as genetic, environmental or autoimmune factors, should also be studied. Closer collaboration between epidemiologists, microbiologists, immunologists, geneticists, environmental scientists, veterinarians, entomologists, clinicians and social scientists is needed to identify the main agents that may be causing these silent infections, to determine the origin of strains and to measure their impact on society. A new multi-directional approach is crucial to expanding the field of research and moving forward. Likewise, patients and physicians must come together to advance care and research together.

Three French associations supporting victims of Lyme Disease have understood this well. That is how in 2015 France Lyme, Lympact and the Relais de Lyme decided to create, together with doctors and researchers, the French Federation against Vector-borne Tick Diseases (FFMVT) with the slogan: 'Patients, doctors, researchers, together'. Unity is strength.

For the sick, I have sworn to myself to continue fighting until the day chronic Lyme and associated diseases are officially recognised in France and the green flag of Lyme recognition flies on Strasbourg University Hospital (where the National Reference Centre for Borreliosis is located).

However, the battle is not yet won because, as Max Planck, Nobel Prize winner in physics in 1918, said: 'A new truth, in science, never succeeds in triumphing by convincing adversaries and bringing them to see the light, but rather because, finally, these adversaries die, and a new generation grows up, to whom this truth is familiar'. It is a pity, because I do not wish for the deaths of my colleagues, many of whom are friends as well as being excellent doctors.

As Richard Buckminster Fuller proclaimed (the man in the United States who developed and improved the architectural concept of the 'geodesic dome' invented by Walther Bauersfeld): 'You don't change things by fighting existing reality. To change something, build a new model that will make the old one obsolete'.

For Charles Nicolle, borrelioses were the 'diseases of the future'. For him, this perspective was intimately linked to a profound conviction: 'Knowledge of infectious diseases teaches men that they are brothers and that they stand in solidarity'.

Four main principles should drive this redeployment, in continuity with the dynamics suggested above:

1. There is 'one health', with animals and humans sharing the same environment, including the microbial environment.
2. Henle-Koch's postulate ('one microbe, one disease') is outdated. There is not only one cause to an illness related to an infection. There may be several microbes involved (bacteria, parasites, fungi, viruses), as well as genetic and environmental factors.
3. The medical community must learn, with the help of researchers, to no longer simply treat the signs and symptoms of many chronic diseases, but to search for their causes in order to propose curative treatments that lead to prolonged remission and even cure in the most favourable cases. Hidden infections, or 'crypto-infections,' really are an important part of these hidden causes.
4. Cancer research should include the infectious dimension of cancer.

To paraphrase another comment by Charles Nicolle, 'crypto infections are and will be the constant companions of our existence. Let's learn to decrypt them. Long live crypto-infectiology and especially long live the sick!'

Chapter 12

Towards a global recognition of chronic Lyme disease

Scientific evidence and lack of good clinical research

Since the publication of the French version of my book in January 2017 scientific evidence demonstrating the existence of chronic Lyme disease has been growing. The fact that blood tests for Lyme disease are not reliable is now well established and increasingly recognised. Since the report of the European Centre for Disease Prevention and Control (ECDC, April 2016 – see page 253), new data have been published, confirming the poor sensitivity of Lyme blood tests. An excellent meta-analysis was published by Cook and Puri in 2016.[61] The mean sensitivity (all tests) is 59.5% (30.6% to 86.2%), far from the 100% still heralded by some experts and laboratories. However, clinical studies using a good methodology and taking into account the huge experience of Lyme-literate medical doctors, are still lacking. Having reviewed what clinical studies there are, there is not a single randomised study to evaluate a really lengthy (four months minimum) antibiotic treatment for chronic Lyme disease. It is amazing to note that this kind of project, which should be a priority, is not funded.

The French National Academy of Medicine

I was invited to participate in a Lyme disease meeting at the French National Academy of Medicine. At that time, the president of the Academy, due to my long experience in evidence-based medicine and in public health, wanted me to become a member of this noble institution. He asked me to give lectures. The first one on Lyme disease in 2015 was in a small room with the infectious disease group of Academicians. This talk was well received. The second one on tuberculosis in June 2016 was in a plenary session and was also appreciated by the audience. Then, on 20 September 2016, I gave a talk on Lyme in a plenary session. Usually, few people from the public attend the plenary sessions of the Academy. That day, the balcony, reserved for the public (the Academicians being seated in the main floor area) was packed full of patients, Lyme doctors and journalists.

I presented evidence-based data on the poor reliability of blood tests, the persistence of infection despite short-term antibiotic treatment and the role of co-infections, as I had done during my previous talk. My slides were full of references supporting this evidence. When the time came for the questions, Professor Marc Gentilini, a retired chief of department of tropical and infectious diseases and former president of the Academy, was shifting around in his chair and asked to speak. His response was violent. He ordered me to retract immediately. As I kept my cool and carried on smiling, he said that I had given an irrational talk. He then accused me of being a terrorist. The hundreds of witnesses, patients, doctors and journalists, were shocked and loud boos came from the balcony. After my calm and firm answers, loud applause resonated under the dome. Gentilini's face turned pale.

Several journalists kept a record of this lamentable event. Many people who had been there suggested I sue for public defamation, but I didn't, out of respect for the former career of this old man who had been a pioneer when, at the beginning of the AIDS epidemic, he was fighting against his colleagues for the recognition of HIV as the cause of disease. It was funny when soon after the Academy meeting, a weekly newspaper in Alsace wrote an article comparing me to Galileo in front of the court of inquisition, where he was asked to retract and to recognise that it was the Sun which was revolving around the Earth. In the title of the article was Galileo's famous sentence about the Earth, 'and still it moves'. The scene has been immortalised by the American cartoonist, David Skidmore, the author of *Lyme Loonies*. I am represented as a refugee on top of the Eiffel tower brandishing the French flag, like the torch of the Statue of Liberty, while people from the ground are shouting 'terrorist' or 'Galileo' or 'Lyme disease witchery'. Some German colleagues who call me 'the lighthouse' congratulated me about this cartoon.

This event has been mentioned by the journalist/writer Marie Pierre Samitier in her book *Le Mystère Borrelia* (in a sweetened formulation), and in one of the reports given to the Special rapporteurs of the United Nations by the Ad Hoc Committee for Health Equity in ICD11 Borreliosis code (discussed below) as an example of the anti-Lyme lobby attitude, and the event is also mentioned by Jenna Luché-Thayer in her book *$lyme*. I was happy to receive warm support from some Academicians who told me in private that the way I was treated was scandalous. Professor Pierre Godeau, a great physician, came to see me at the end of the Academy session to tell me how he had been shocked. Others prefer to remain anonymous. Since this event, several Academicians have told me to continue my fight and some have written to me, asking for my support for people in their family with chronic Lyme!

The Ad Hoc Committee for Health Equity in ICD11 Borreliosis code

In 2017, I met Jenna Luché-Thayer, who is a former Senior Advisor to the United Nations and US government, with 32 years' experience in human rights across 42 nations. She took the lead in a global coalition of physicians and researchers named the Ad Hoc Committee for Health Equity in ICD11 Borreliosis code. We had meetings in Geneva at the World Health Organization (WHO) and with United Nations Special Rapporteurs and other UN officials. In 2017 and 2018, we met two Special Rapporteurs of the UN. Our two reports, now published, helped to open these doors.[14, 15] They document how the absence of adequate diagnostic codes, the absence of reliable diagnostic tests and the rejection by physicians of millions of patients is no longer acceptable and amounts to the violation of human rights on all continents.

During these meetings, I met Dr Kenneth B Liegner and I realised that he was a great pioneer who spoke on the human rights violations of patients with tick borne diseases. Dr Liegner has published a book that reviews 25 years of 'Lyme wars'. I also met Dr Sin Hang Lee, who developed PCR diagnostic tests in collaboration with the CDC and eventually had a $57 million lawsuit underway against the CDC for interfering with patents access to his validated technology. Unfortunately, he lost his fight for justice.

The WHO's International Classification of Diseases (ICD) version 10 (ICD10), recognised only four codes for Lyme disease, without any recognition of the numerous clinical forms of the disease, especially those linked to the chronicity of infection. For syphilis, the other 'great imitator' disease, the number of codes is huge. Our efforts had results. In June 2018, the WHO released the revised version of ICD, ICD11, that added several new codes for Lyme, including a code for Lyme dementia and a code for the maternal-foetal transmission or congenital Lyme disease. The need for the code for congenital Lyme has since been disputed, creating a global demand to protect the code and recognise the life-threatening complications of congenital Lyme disease.

Professors in Europe

Professors of medicine fighting for the recognition of chronic Lyme disease are very rare in Europe (and in the rest of the world). Some have been threatened and others persecuted. In Norway, Professor Carl Morten Laane, microbiologist at the University of Bergen came under attack because, despite several warnings, he continued to present his data showing the persistence of *Borrelia* under the microscope. Since the conference I wrote about in Chapter 7 (see page 128) he has been fired by his university and one of his publications has been withdrawn from a scientific journal.

I have met Professor Jack Lambert, of Scottish origin who worked in the United States in the HIV-AIDS domain and is now professor of infectious diseases in Dublin, Ireland. I was happy to meet him and to find an excellent university colleague, physician and researcher, to work with on a scientific basis. Jack is doing a fantastic job and recently opened a specialised centre in Ireland for educating patients and general practitioners (GPs) about Lyme and other crypto-infections. In response to his establishing this 'education and research centre' focused on educating the public and GPs to be better able to recognise tick-borne infections early, a number of his 'colleagues' in Ireland (all members of the IDSA 'clique' – see page 107) have tried to sabotage this initiative. So here we go again with the IDSA mantra: there are no ticks, there is no Lyme, patients are making up their illness, it is a rare disease that is easy to diagnose and easy to treat. And for those who do not get better with a short course of treatment, but who do on a longer course of antibiotics, it is a placebo effect… as there is no such thing as 'chronic Lyme'!

Not much has changed in the rhetoric of the IDSA Lyme clique over the last decade, but actually worldwide, a lot has changed that those in IDSA need to start waking up to. As attacks continue both on doctors and indeed patient groups, it is not surprising that other professors in Europe who believe in the cause don't want to step forward, fearing the establishment and the consequences of speaking out

The need for a multidisciplinary approach

In many countries, it is difficult to develop new diagnostic tests. Some groups of experts have a monopoly on deciding which test is valid or not, and which research should be developed and funded or not. In France, the National Reference Centre (NRC) for Borreliosis in Strasbourg has a monopoly on the validation of tests and on decisions to develop new diagnostic strategies. No other human biological lab has invested in research on borreliosis. Thus, new tests such as polymerase chain reactions (PCRs), which are not developed by the NRC, are blocked. If sensitive enough, PCR would eliminate the problem of non-reliable blood tests. Veterinary biological labs which develop new PCRs for animals are denounced by the health authorities or the Medicines Agency (ANSM), which is also in charge of medical products and devices, if they do any work for humans. As our Minister of Health, Professor Agnès Buzyn, asked the ANSM to review and validate all the blood tests for *Borrelia* marketed in France, I wondered how this agency could verify the quality of calibration of the test kits, since, as acknowledged by the European Centre for Diseases Prevention and Control (ECDC), it is almost impossible to calibrate Lyme serology, due to the lack of well-defined populations of patients and healthy controls.

In July 2018, I asked for a meeting with ANSM's experts to be informed about their method. Evaluation is made by testing healthy blood donor samples. The following response astonished me: the 'gold-standard' to evaluate all tests is the 'official' two-tier blood test from the NRC – yet there is published evidence that this technique is no good. When I told them that it was hugely biased, they were embarrassed and answered that, even if I was right, they had no other means of performing this evaluation. Other techniques, such as quantitative dosage of antigens, should be developed. Progress cannot come from a single lab. Synergies and competition are needed to move forward, in a multidisciplinary approach. For example, we need to work more closely with immunologists. Some of them are currently working on borreliosis and the immune response. It is now established that *Borreliae* may induce immunosuppression. So, some co-infections could be opportunistic infections, as seen in AIDS. Researchers are developing new immunologic markers that could help with diagnosis. As discussed in Chapter 9, persistent viruses are probably involved in many chronic conditions. Some viruses are known to persist in the body, as we saw. In addition to the well-known viruses such as hepatitis viruses, HIV, EBV, CMV, herpes simplex and varicella-zoster, recent data show that tick-borne encephalitis virus (TBEV), Zika virus, West Nile virus and Powassan virus may persist. In the United States, a high proportion of patients with chronic Lyme are infected with the Powassan virus. Some physicians suspect endogenous retroviruses, harboured by all animals or humans, of being responsible for some chronic disorders. Serious virologic studies are needed.

French health authorities launch a national plan

Following the creation of the French Federation against Tick-borne Diseases (FFMVT) in 2015, grouping three associations of patients and supporters, a college of physicians and researchers and a scientific council, advocacy has been based on scientific arguments and medical literature. I was elected chairman of the scientific council of the FFMVT in 2015. The analysis of published data showed that the evidence was on our side. This initiative increased our visibility and led to better consideration by the media and politicians, with a now positive image.

In September 2016, the French health authorities, the Minister of Health, the Director General for Health, and the Haute Autorité de Santé (High Authority for Health) acknowledged that Lyme disease presents a great problem in public health and that diagnostic tests and treatment strategies should be revised. The Minister for Health, Marisol Touraine, recognised publicly that many chronic Lyme patients have been abandoned and rejected by the health system. As mentioned earlier, she decided in September 2016 to launch a National plan. Five strategic axes were defined:

1. Improve the surveillance of vectors and the measures against ticks in a 'WHO one health' approach (humans/animals).
2. Enhance surveillance and prevention of tick-borne diseases.
3. Improve and standardise the management of patients.
4. Improve diagnostic tests.
5. Develop research on tick-borne diseases.

Unfortunately, as we'll see, this plan was blocked.

When the French plan was launched I met Professor Agnès Buzyn, who was President of HAS. I had crossed her path a long time before when she had been a trainee in the department where I was working. The HAS was charged with creating a working group to look at the management of patients. In 2017 Agnès Buzyn was appointed as Minister of Health. She resigned in 2020, at the beginning of the Covid-19 epidemic in Europe.

I participated in the Strategic Axis 3 working group on improving and standardising the management of patients. It was a multi-disciplinary group of experts, under the auspices of HAS. The group included representatives of medical societies with physicians from several specialties including representatives of the French Infectious Diseases Society (SPILF), microbiologists, general practitioners, the National Reference Centre (NRC) for Borreliosis, patients and Lyme doctors from the FFMVT. Jérôme Salomon, who was professor of infectious and tropical diseases in my department and who had always helped me in the management of chronic Lyme patients, was co-chair of this working group. Later on, in January 2018, he was appointed as Director General for Health at the Ministry. The group was composed of pro- and anti- chronic Lyme disease experts, and they arrived at a final consensus and wrote the new French recommendations entitled *Recommendation of Good Practice for Lyme Disease and other Tick-borne Diseases*.

The *Recommendation* is made up of two parts: a short text (the recommendations themselves) which are theoretically consensual, and a longer text, the *Argumentaire scientifique* (scientific review) including medical references. Differing opinions could be expressed in the longer text. For clinical forms of Lyme disease, blood tests are recommended, but a positive result is not mandatory to make the diagnosis. The text recognises officially a new syndrome called SPPT, *syndrome polymorphe persistant après une possible piqûre de tique,* which means 'Persistent polymorphic syndrome possibly due to a tick bite'. SPPT may be due to Lyme, co-infections and/or other factors. The link with a tick bite does not need to be established. The blood test for Lyme or co-infections may be negative. SPPT was already mentioned in the report written by the High Council for Public Health (HCSP) in 2014. SPPT is close to the PTLDS (post-treatment Lyme disease syndrome), but without the need to prove a Lyme diagnosis or for previous antibiotic treatment.

PTLDS does not specify whether ongoing signs and symptoms are infectious or post-infectious in nature, while SPPT postulates ongoing untreated infection or partially treated infection that should be treated with antibiotics. The diagnosis of SPPT is mainly clinical.

In cases of SPPT, every general practitioner can prescribe, after exclusion of other diagnoses, an empiric antibiotic treatment as a diagnostic trial, to assess response to one month of doxycycline. A response to treatment confirms the bacterial origin of this condition. The initial response may be a worsening of symptoms (the Jarisch-Herxheimer reaction or 'Herx' as discussed earlier). There is also the possibility of prescribing antimicrobial drugs beyond one month, without limitations on duration of treatment or choice of drugs. The general practitioner must collaborate with an expert hospital centre (five national referral centres and additional centres under their supervision). Centres will be appointed by the Ministry for Health after a national call. Expert centres should have representatives of Lyme patients in their steering committee. Treatments and outcomes must be registered in order to collect data for research (observational research, cohorts). Some volunteer patients will be included in clinical trials (for the evaluation of new diagnostic tests, randomised trials...). GPs are free to choose the expert centre they wish to use (it would not be mandatory to choose the regional one). As mentioned above, it appeared later on that the centres set up by the Ministry of Health were under the control of anti-Lyme doctors.

It was intended that, after the release of the Recommendations, persecution of doctors treating Lyme patients should stop. Expert centres would receive funding for manpower and material resources, in order to register the data.

The problem was that these new recommendations were immediately attacked. After the final agreement, colleagues who had worked within the group and agreed until the final meeting on the consensual text, refused to sign it and launched attacks and lobbied to obtain the support of medical societies. Several medical societies (of specialists and general practitioners) asked for a boycott of the text. Modifications to the text were made by the French Infectious Disease Society (SPILF) and by the NRC for Borreliosis in Strasbourg, without the agreement of the members from the FFMVT.

These alterations were not consensual at all. The two-tier blood test strategy was added afterwards without the agreement of the whole group: Elisa first, and if positive, Western blot after, as before. An annex (Annex 3) on 'The performance of diagnostic tests' was added. In the table of this annex, blood tests were presented as very accurate, with sensitivities as high as 100% for some clinical forms of the condition (arthritis and acrodermatitis chronicum atrophicans). This misconduct from the anti-Lyme experts of the group was a violation of the usual procedure of an official working group yet the college of HAS maintained the alterations in the final text. These modifications do not have a strong impact, since a positive blood test result is no longer mandatory, so, despite this shameful violation, the new French recommendations are a form of progress.

At the end of 2020, the fight continues as it appears that the expert centres are not being established according to the Recommendations (e.g. participation of patients and Lyme doctors). Planned by the authorities to appease the Lyme issue, these recommendations triggered unprecedented violent and irrational attacks, in the name of science but not based on science, from the anti-Lyme lobbies ('go too far…') and surprisingly from some patients and physicians ('don't go far enough…'). Despite these polemics, followed in the media, the Recommendations were finally officially released in July 2018 by the HAS (see page 323 for a link to this document).

These recommendations were intended to protect physicians against persecution. However, in June 2018, the French

Infectious Disease Society (SPILF) called on all physicians and pharmacists to denounce Lyme doctors, still considered to be charlatans. Since then the number of persecutions has increased from both Social Security and the Order of Physicians, and some pharmacists now refuse to provide drugs for Lyme and co-infection treatments.

In 2020, the situation is worsening. Reference centres refuse to follow the official guidelines of the HAS. For the patients, it is a betrayal and a violation of health democracy. The government is under pressure from the anti-Lyme lobbies which ignore science and are influenced by the French Academy of Medicine.

Fortunately, more and more deputies and senators support the chronic Lyme patients and their doctors. They have written amendments, but currently, these texts have been rejected by the Ministry of Health and by the Ministry of Higher Education and Research. At the end of 2019, Agnès Buzyn, as Minister of Health, rejected a project to fund Lyme research, which had been written by MPs. She said 'no' in front of those MPs at the National Assembly. And the political obstruction remains strong and persistent. On 10 November 2020, the National Assembly persisted in the denial and voted to reject a budget for research into Lyme disease that had been requested by 80 MPs. The demand for funding was strongly attacked by Frédérique Vidal, Minister for Higher Education and Research. After the hopes raised by the 2016 national plan, patients have never been so distressed.

Phytotherapy, a strategy for the future

In 2018, I met Professor Ying Zhang, a microbiologist in Baltimore at the Johns Hopkins University, who is one of the leading researchers on the evaluation of drugs for the persistent forms of *Borrelia*. I have cited his main publications in the reference section of this book (page 319). He is increasingly working on herbal treatments and finding very interesting results. Some natural products, such as oregano, may be more active on bacteria than antibiotics. Ying Zhang came to France at the end of October 2018 for a closed meeting at the Pasteur Institute in Paris and was invited to the annual scientific meeting of the French Federation against Tick-borne Diseases (FFMVT) in Montpellier. We had discussions about the amazing antimicrobial power of some plants and agreed that research should be developed in this field. It is a priority since new antibiotics are not being developed anymore, except for some rare drugs. In 2020 Yin Zhang went back to China, his native country.

When I spoke publicly about my support for phytotherapy, I was attacked. Opponents said that the effect of plants was a placebo effect, or that plants were dangerous and that, in any case, their efficacy had never been demonstrated. Given this response, I really wanted to participate in clinical trials demonstrating the efficacy of some herbal extracts and took part in two big clinical trials, following the good clinical practices recommended by WHO. The studies were conducted in Africa and showed that the whole plant *Artemisia* is more effective than chemical comparators for the treatment of schistosomiasis and of malaria.

The leader of the *Artemisia* projects is Dr Lucile Cornet-Vernet, a wonderfully energetic and enthusiastic woman. We worked with a very talented physician from Congo-Kinshasa, Dr Jérôme Munyangi. Both studies used a double-blind method. For schistosomiasis, 800 patients were included, and for malaria, 1000 patients. The major problem with these studies was the difficulty in getting them funded. As you cannot patent a plant, manufacturers do not invest in research into herbal medicines that would not allow a return on investment.

These studies were published but our articles were strongly attacked, presumably because the efficacy of *Artemisia* may ruin the potential benefits of drugs or vaccines. There were small imperfections in the databases used, due to the difficult conditions in which the studies were carried out. We informed the medical journal that published our articles and gave the databases to our detractors to convince them that the imperfections did not change the statistics, nor the results. Despite these proofs of good faith, aggressive lobbying resulted in the retraction of the articles.

Deniers of Lyme disease are losing the battle but continue to fight on

Some deniers are still saying that persistent forms of *Borrelia* do not exist, though it is proven in the medical literature that they do.[153, 208] In France, some experts, under the influence of the National Reference Centre (NRC) for Borreliosis and the National Academy of Medicine say and write in the media that all patients are cured after a three-week course of antibiotics and that there is not a single reference published showing that *Borrelia* may persist in the body after a short-term antibiotic treatment.

How can such misinformation still be spread? Numerous articles show that persistent signs and symptoms after 'classical' (short) antibiotic treatment are observed in 16–62% of patients.[29, 57, 79, 81, 172, 173, 207, 210] When you present this information to deniers, they tell you that the clinical data are not strong and that we need bacteriological data. So, here are the bacteriological data. The persistence of *Borreliae* was first proven in animals, even after several months of antibiotic treatment in the following articles: Straubinger et al, 1997; Straubinger, 2000; Embers et al, 2004; Hodzic et al, 2008; Barthold et al, 2010; Embers et al, 2012; Embers et al, 2017.

The deniers will then tell you that results in animals are not representative of human infection. (Why are they not?) The following are the results in humans. The persistence of *Borreliae* has been shown in humans after antibiotic treatment of erythema migrans in these published articles: Hunfeld et al, 2005; Strle et al, 1993; Weber et al, 1993. In a later stage of the disease, the persistence of *Borreliae* is proven since these bacteria can be isolated by culture or PCR in humans after antibiotic treatment of chronic Lyme disease as shown by: Haupl et al, 1993; Lawrence et al, 1995; Lee et al, 2014; Masters et al, 1994; Murgia and Cinco, 2004; Oksi et al, 1998; Oksi et al, 1999; Pfister et al, 1991; Phillips et al, 1998; Preac-Mursic et al, 1996; Preac-Mursic et al, 1993; Preac-Mursic et al, 1989; Schmidli et al, 1988; and Middleveen et al, 2018.

These numerous publications clearly demonstrate the clinical persistence of signs and symptoms, validating the existence of chronic Lyme disease, and the microbiological persistence of *Borreliae*. In the study by Oksi and collaborators, published in 1999, the culture and PCR for *Borrelia* was positive in 40% of patients who relapsed.[173] In the study by Middleveen and collaborators published in 2018, PCRs from patients and from control healthy subjects were analysed using a double-blind method, in three different laboratories.[15] Results of PCR were compared with microscopic examination and culture. In October 2018, Garg et al published a paper showing that varied co-infections existed in 65% of patients: *Borrelia burgdorferi s.s., Borrelia garinii* and *Borrelia afzelii* (spirochetes and persistent forms), *Babesia microti, Bartonella henselae, Brucella abortus, Ehrlichia chaffeensis, Rickettsia akari, Chlamydia pneumoniae, Chlamydia trachomatis, Mycoplasma pneumonia,* and viruses, such as tick-borne encephalitis virus (TBEV), Coxsackie A16, CMV, EBV, and parvovirus B19.[95]

This shows how urgent it is to abandon the postulate of: one microbe, one disease. It is interesting to note that, in 2016, the presence of *Chamydiae* in ticks and in the human skin after tick bite had already been reported by Hokynar et al.[112]

In the United States, the website of the National Guidelines Clearinghouse (NGC), which had withdrawn the obsolete IDSA guidelines in 2016, posted the ILADS recommendations.

However, in July 2018, funding for the NGC ended. The 2018 Report to Congress by the Tick-borne Disease Working Group, organised in the United States by the US Department of Health and Human Services, recognised the lack of good diagnostic tests, the absence of good clinical trials to evaluate treatments, the persistence of signs and symptoms, and the possibility of the persistence of bacteria. The report insisted on the fact that co-infections had been neglected and that we did not have good diagnostic tests for them. It also acknowledged that there had not been significant research for decades and insisted on the need to fund research. After all this scientific evidence, deniers should not be allowed anymore to say that chronic Lyme disease does not exist, and worse, to misinform physicians all around the world.

In Europe, National Reference Centres (NRC) for Borreliosis and the myopic 'learned societies' who cannot read, or don't want to read, scientific publications remain completely aligned with the obsolete 2006 IDSA recommendations, which are not recognised in the United States anymore. IDSA still has strong support in Europe through EUCALB and now ESGBOR, the new working group on borreliosis organised by the European Society of Clinical Microbiology and Infectious Diseases (ESCMID). While most health authorities continue to follow these unreliable sources, politicians from all European countries, seeing the despair of more and more patients every day, are sounding the alarm.

However, misinformation continues to spread. In June 2017, Karen Rowan wrote a very misleading article saying that 'unproven treatments' for chronic Lyme disease could kill the patients. Rare cases of deaths are reported, but in all the cases, death was due to a complication of a central intravenous catheter (a thin tube allowing infusions directly into the pulmonary artery, near the heart), and not related to antibiotics. The consequence was that many medical journals spread the fake news that it was now 'proven' that prolonged antibiotic treatment of Lyme was dangerous and might kill. In fact, without exception, there are no indications for use of such catheters for Lyme patients.

In September 2018, infectious disease physicians from a Parisian hospital, followers of Professor Marc Gentilini (Haddad et al, 2018), published an astonishing paper in *Clinical Infectious Diseases* saying that less than 10% of possible chronic Lyme patients really had Lyme (the others were psychiatric or had another disease: chronic fatigue syndrome, fibromyalgia, autoimmune disease, etc) and among these 'confirmed' cases, antibiotic failure was observed in more than 80% of them. The history of a tick bite was mandatory for the diagnosis, although it had been published that three quarters of proven Lyme patients don't recall any tick-bite. The official blood test had to be positive (Elisa and Western blot), though the unreliability of these tests had been published in the scientific literature. It is sad to read these 'results' but it illustrates exactly the way patients are treated by the physicians who are not Lyme literate. The final result of their management in this paper was that 20% of the patients were cured among less than 10% of 'confirmed' cases. That represents two patients or less cured among 100 patients. That is a shame when we know that we can improve the medical condition or cure around 80% of the patients when they are treated by Lyme-literate doctors. In Haddad et al's 2018 article, treatment failure was defined as being when patients still showed persistent signs and symptoms despite four weeks of antibiotic therapy. It was a major bias of the study.

Borrelia has the capacity to persist (in its round form or when located within biofilms), and co-infections, including parasitic infections, were not looked for nor discussed. The so-called 'therapeutic failure' of a short one-month therapy was confused, in many cases, with clinical exacerbation reactions (Jarish-Herxheimer reactions), which may occur during the first days of treatment but also one, two or three weeks later and may oscillate during weeks and sometimes months during treatment, as I explained in Chapter 8. Fortunately, our robust reply to *Clinical Infectious Diseases* was published on 21 November 2018.[13]

Another example of denial promotion was a paper published in December 2018 in *Médecine et Maladies Infectieuses*, the journal of the French Infectious Disease Society (SPILF) (Eldin et al, 2018). The authors were Didier Raoult from Marseille, some of his colleagues, and representatives of SPILF and the French NRC for Borreliosis. They compiled several sets of guidelines published around the world since 2006.

These guidelines were generally wholesale copies of the obsolete, now withdrawn recommendations of IDSA, which were not based on evidence in the first place. These guidelines ignored many recent scientific publications without any updating. They rejected the guidelines of the German Borreliosis Society which are the only ones to recognise the chronic form of the disease. The recent report of the US Department of Health and Human Services, which conducted a complete review of the literature, was not even mentioned. Four of the authors of this paper participated in the French HAS working group and contributed to the writing of the new French Recommendations published in June 2018 yet these official French recommendations were not cited. Despite all these biases and omissions, the authors concluded that experts from all over the world agreed that chronic Lyme did not exist, and that the two-tier blood test was reliable. That was pure misinformation, if not pure propaganda.

Global collaboration is the way forward

A young American Lyme patient, Olivia Goodreau, created with her parents the LivLyme Foundation. In September 2018, her mother Holiday Goodreau, invited me to give a talk in Denver on the new French Recommendations. I was able to meet experts of the working group on Lyme and co-infections established by the US Department of Human and Health Services. I could speak with Dr Richard Horowitz, whom I had known well for a long time and Kristen Honey, vice-chair of the group. Their recent report to Congress and their subcommittee reports described many issues the French national plan tried to address. Thus, France and the United States have followed pathways that should meet for the good.

This accumulation of evidence and political support in many countries makes me think that the 'Berlin wall' of denial is not far from collapsing. In the Decision 1082/2013 of the European Parliament and the Council of the European Union passed in 2013, Lyme borreliosis was deemed as a 'Serious cross-border threat to life', 'life-threatening or otherwise serious hazard to health ...' and a disease which may necessitate coordination at Union level. High level experts supported this alert: the European Centre for Disease Prevention and Control (ECDC) published in August 2017 a handbook and manual *ECDC Tool for the Prioritisation of Infectious Disease Threats*. Lyme borreliosis was listed among the 30 most threatening diseases in public health importance (there was no ranking of the 30 diseases). Thanks to the brilliant work of the Belgian European MP, Frédérique Ries and her team, on the 15 November 2018, the European Parliament, with a unanimous vote, passed a Resolution asking Member States to act on recognition and research for Lyme disease and co-infections.

Fearing to lose control of the situation, some physicians, afraid of change, become more radicalised. Professor François Bricaire, member of the National Academy of Medicine and follower of Marc Gentilini, had previously been quite open-minded, since he was the co-author of the 2014 HCSP report, which created the concept of SPPT (persistent polymorphic syndrome possibly due to a tick bite), diagnosed clinically, even if Lyme blood tests were negative and recommending empiric antibiotic treatment as a diagnostic test. However, in

2018 he wrote and said in several media outlets that SPPT was a bad concept invented by people who are not scientifically minded. His follower, Professor Eric Caumes, organised with the French Infectious Diseases Society (SPILF), the NRC for Borreliosis and several learned societies a working group to write 'recommendations' to suppress SPPT. Two articles were published in 2019,[92, 117] but have no value since they were not created using a valid methodology and were written without the input of patients. Thus, they should not be entitled 'guidelines'; they are only 'expert advice', and not recognised officially.

The same story happened in the United States where IDSA, upset to have been kept out of the official US working group, published online a draft of new unofficial 'recommendations'. On both sides of the pond, they declare that their new advice is 'evidence based'. In fact, the experts' advice, from the SPILF in France and from the IDSA in the USA, does not take into account numerous international published articles. For the patients, these texts are worse than the 2006 guidelines, either American or French. In September 2019, the Ad Hoc Patient and Physician Coalition protested against the IDSA Lyme 'guidelines' and has continued to gather steam throughout the world. Lorraine Johnson of *LymeDisease.org* and Dr Betty Maloney of ILADS wrote a very well referenced rebuttal of the 'guidelines', and so far, 88 organisations in 12 countries have endorsed the coalition's rebuttal. Countries represented include: the USA, Canada, Australia, France, Germany, Great Britain, the Netherlands, Belgium, Latvia, Spain, Poland and Czechia.

Fearing the judgement of history, some deniers are starting to retract…

First of all IDSA. In a recent article published in October 2018, Schutzer, with several members of the IDSA Lyme clique published an article saying that Lyme blood tests were not so good (at least for quite early forms of the disease) and that PCRs could be interesting to develop.[203] I was so happy to read that, given decades of saying that antibody blood testing was perfect and PCR for Lyme or co-infections was not useful.

A theory, known as the 'amber theory', argues that spirochetes that can be seen under the microscope in patients' tissue are dead bacteria, in a fossil state.[243] Positive PCR for *Borreliae* could be false-positive tests amplifying the debris of nucleic acids. Eva Sapi and her team demonstrated that *Borrelia* may remain alive within biofilms.[196]

The second example of deniers in retreat is the director of the French National Reference Centre (NRC) for Borreliosis in Strasbourg, Professor Benoît Jaulhac. He was co-author of an article by Robinot et al published in December 2018 in the journal *Blood*. The title of the article is 'Chronic *Borrelia burgdorferi* infection triggers NKT lymphomagenesis'. Yes, you have read the title correctly! When, the year before, I and my colleagues had worked with Benoît Jaulhac in the HAS working group, we were not allowed to pronounce these iconoclastic words. The word 'chronic' was forbidden! I now congratulate Professor Jaulhac for his open mind and welcome him into the chronic Lyme world.

The NRC in Strasbourg represented by Benoît Jaulhac, and Didier Raoult's team in Marseille published an article in February 2019 entitled 'Values of diagnostic tests for the various species of spirochetes' (Eldin et al, 2019). They wrote that no diagnostic test was perfect, and that the physician must take into account the clinical and epidemiological context when suspecting the disease. It was really good to see these facts written by persons who had previously always said that the available blood tests were excellent tests.

The growing awareness of Lyme disease demands the pharmaceutical industry improves diagnostic testing, and treaments, for Lyme and its co-infections. Pharmaceutical manufacturers, most of whom have ignored the Lyme field over three decades, are back in play. New vaccines and new diagnostic tests are being developed. It is not clear that vaccines, which would be limited to a small number of *Borrelia* species and not active in preventing co-infections will be a real solution, but research could improve the concept. This urgent need for research and development encourages recognition of chronic Lyme disease and, more generally, the need for more knowledge in the huge field of crypto-infections.

The publication in May 2019 of the book *Bitten* by Kris Newby, revealing secret archives from Willy Burgdorfer, will probably have a positive impact on political decisions. Kris Newby declared in her book that she had digital copies of the lab archives showing that Willy Burgdorfer and his colleagues modified by mutation several species of *Borrelia*, *Rickettsia*, especially *Rickettsia helvetica* (called by Burgdorfer the 'Swiss agent'). *Babesia* and viruses... to obtain tick-borne biological weapons. The author also related the human experiments conducted on 'volunteers' in 'Operation Whitecoat' cited earlier in this book (page 91). These 'volunteers' were in fact conscientious objectors who wanted to escape the Vietnam war. After the release of the book, the US House of Representatives called for an investigation into whether the spread of Lyme disease had its roots in a Pentagon experiment in weaponising ticks. In July 2019, the House approved an amendment instructing the Defense Department's Inspector General to conduct a review, that is still ongoing at the time of writing.

Fortunately in France, the media coverage of Lyme disease is growing. The fact that more and more journalists take time to read scientific data, instead of following fake information from the learned societies, and support the cause of patients is a major breakthrough. Of course, this does not please SPILF (the French Infectious Diseases Society). In November 2019, Pascal et al published in the *European Journal of Public Health* an article complaining about my excess coverage in the French media. I'm called 'WB' in their text, standing not for 'Western blot' but for 'whistle blower'. I feel honoured by this publication written against me, since I consider their complaint to be a tribute. I'm proud to be a whistle blower.

All the scientific data, the political debate, the media coverage, the recent funding for research in the USA, the return of pharmaceutical companies to the field and, unfortunately for the patients, the dramatic increase of the Lyme pandemic will inevitably lead to the global recognition of chronic Lyme disease and other chronic crypto-infections. A new specialty is emerging. The First European Conference on Crypto-infections took place in Dublin, Ireland, on 31 May – 1 June 2019. Due to travel restrictions imposed during the Covid-19 epidemic, the second conference was realised by videoconference on 26–27 September 2020. Long live crypto-infectiology!

References

Scientific articles

Author's articles

1. Borgermans L, Perronne C, Balicer R, Plasek O, Obsomer V. Lyme disease: time for a new approach? *British Medical Journal* 2015; 351. doi: 10.1136/bmj.h6520.
2. Clarissou J, Song A, Bernede C, Guillemot D, Dinh A, Ader F, Perronne C, Salomon J. Efficacy of a long-term antibiotic treatment in patients with a chronic tick associated poly-organic syndrome (TAPOS). *Médecine et Maladies Infectieuses* 2009; 39(2): 108–115.
3. Davido B, Bouchand F, Calin R, Makhloufi S, Lagrange A, Senard O, Perronne C, Villart M, Salomon J, Dinh A. High rates of off-label use in antibiotic prescriptions in a context of dramatic resistance increase: A prospective study in a tertiary hospital. *International Journal Antimicrobial Agents* 2016; 47(6): 490–494.
4. Franck M, Ghozzi R, Pajaud J, Lawson-Hogban NE, Mas M, Lacout A, Perronne C. *Borrelia miyamotoi*; 43 cases diagnosed in France by real-time PCR in patients with persistent polymorphic signs and symptoms. *Front Med* 2020. doi: 10.3389/fmed.2020.00055.
5. Galpérine T, Lacout A, Marcy PY, Perronne C. Favorable outcome after treatment using antibiotics and hydroxychloroquine in a patient with tulor necrosis factor receptor-associated periodic syndrome: A 7-year follow-up. *Journal of Global Infectious Diseases* 2020; 12: 158-160.
6. Ghez D, Bernard L, Bayou E, Bani-Sadr F, Vallée C, Perronne C. *Bartonella henselae* infection mimicking a splenic lymphoma. *Scandinavian Journal of Infectious Diseases* 2001; 33(12): 935–936.

7. Horowitz RI, Lacout A, Marcy PY, Perronne C. To test or not to test? Laboratory support for the diagnosis of Lyme borreliosis. *Clinical Microbiology Infection* 2018; 24: 210. doi: 10.1016:j.cmi.2017.09.015.
8. Lacout A, Dacher V, El Hajjam M, Marcy PY, Perronne C. Biofilms busters to improve the detection of *Borrelia* using PCR. *Medical Hypotheses* 2018; 112: 4–6. doi: 10.1016/j.mehy.2018.01.005.
9. Lacout A, Mone Y, Franck M, Marcy PY, Mas M, Veas F, Perronne C. Blood cell disruption to significantly improve the *Borrelia* PCR detection sensitivity in borreliosis in humans. *Medical Hypotheses* 2018; 116: 1–3. doi: 10.1016/j.mehy.2018.04.012.
10. Lacout A, Marcy PY, Mas M, Perronne C. Holistic or dedicated approach in Lyme disease? *Clinical Infectious Disease* 2018. doi.org/10.1093/cid/ciy995.
11. Lacout A, Marcy PY, El Hajjam M, Thariat J, Perronne C. Dealing with Lyme disease treatment. *American Journal Medicine* 2017; 130: e221. doi: 10.1016/j.amjmed.2016.12.039.
12. Lacout A, Thariat J, Hajjam ME, Marcy PY, Perronne C. Lyme disease and co-infections: role of adaptative immune system. *Future Microbiology* 2018; 13: 613–615. doi: 10.2217/fmb-2017-0252.
13. Lacout A, El Hajjam M, Marcy PY, Perronne C. The persistent Lyme disease: 'true chronic Lyme disease' rather than 'post-treatment Lyme disease syndrome'. *Journal of Global Infectious Disease* 2018; 10: 170–171. doi: 10.4103:jgid.jgid_152_17.
14. Luché-Thayer J, Ahern H, Bransfield R, et al. The situation of human rights defenders of Lyme and relapsing fever Borreliosis: Edition One: The Ad Hoc Committee for Health Equity in ICD11 Borreliosis Codes. 2018. CreateSpace Independent Publishing Platform, Scotts Valley, California.
15. Luché-Thayer J, Perronne C, Meseko C. Obstruction to treatments meeting international standards for Lyme and relapsing fever borreliosis Patients. *World Academy of Science, Engineering and Technology International Journal of Law and Political Sciences* 2018; 12(6).
16. Perronne C. Lyme disease antiscience. *Lancet Infectious Disease* 2012; 12(5): 361–362.
17. Perronne C. Lyme and associated tick-borne diseases: Global challenges in the context of a public health threat. *Frontiers in Cellular Infectious Microbiology* 2014; 4: 74.

18. Perronne C. Critical review of studies trying to evaluate the treatment of chronic Lyme disease. *Presse Medicale* 2015: 44(7–8): 828–831.
19. Roche-Lanquetot M-O, Ader F, Durand M-C, Carlier R, Defferière H, Dinh A, Herrmann JL, Guillemot D, Perronne C, Salomon J. Results of a prospective standardized study of 30 patients with chronic neurological and cognitive disorders after tick bites (in French). *Médecine et Maladies Infectieuses* 2008; 38(10): 543–548.

Other articles

20. Aase A, Hajdusek O, Oines O, Quarsten H, Wilhemsson P, Herstad TK et al. Validate or falsify: Lessons learned from a microscopy method claimed to be useful for detecting *Borrelia* and *Babesia* organisms in human blood. *Infectious Diseases* 2016; 48(6): 411–419.
21. Afzelius A. Negotiations of the Dermatological Society of Stockholm, *Archive für Dermatologie und Syphilis* 1910; 101: 405–406.
22. Aguero-Rosenfeld ME. Lyme disease: Laboratory issues. *Infectious Diseases Clinical North America* 2008; 22(2): 301–313.
23. Alban PS, Johnson PW, Nelson DR. Serum-starvation-induced changes in protein synthesis and morphology of *Borrelia burgdorferi*. *Microbiology* 2000; 146 (Pt 1): 119–127.
24. Allen HB, Morales D, Jones K, Joshi S. Alzheimer's disease: A novel hypothesis integrating spirochetes, biofilm, and the immune system. *Journal of Neuroinfectious Diseases* 2016; 7(1). doi:10.4172/2314–7326.1000200.
25. American Academy of Pediatrics Steering Committee on Quality Improvement and Management. Classifying recommendations for clinical practice guidelines. *Pediatrics* 2004; 114: 874–877.
26. Ang CW, Notermans DW, Hommes M, Simoons-Smit AM, Herremans T. Large differences between test strategies for the detection of anti-*Borrelia* anti-bodies are revealed by comparing eight ELISAs and five immunoblots. *European Journal Clinical Microbiology Infectious Disease* 2011; 30(8): 1027–1032.
26a. Arshad S, Kilgore P, Chaudhry ZS, Jacobsen G, Wang DD, Huitsing K, et al. Treatment with hydroxychloroquine,

azithromycin, and combination in patients hospitalized with COVID-19. *International Journal of Infectious Diseases* 2020; 97: 396–403. https://doi.org/10.1016/j.ijid.2020.06.099.

27. Arnoud-Meyer C, Stijnen T, Wasser MNJM, Hamming JF, van Bockel JH, Lindeman JHN et al. Doxycycline for stabilization of abdominal aortic aneurysms: A randomized trial. *Annals of Internal Medicine* 2013; 159: 815-823.
28. Assous MV. Laboratory methods for the diagnosis of clinical forms of Lyme borreliosis. *Médecine et Maladies Infectieuses* 2007; 37(7–8): 487–495.
29. Asch ES, Bujak DI, Weiss M, et al. Lyme disease: an infectious and postinfectious syndrome. *Journal of Rheumatology* 1994; 21: 454–461.
30. Auwaerter PG, Bakken JS, Dattwyler RJ, Dumler JS, Halperin JJ, McSweegan E, Nadelman RB, O'Connell S, Shapiro ED, Sood SK, Steere AC, Weinstein A, Wormser GP. Antiscience and ethical concerns associated with advocacy of Lyme disease. *Lancet Infectious Disease* 2011; 11(9): 713–719.
31. Auwaerter PG. Editorial commentary: Life after Lyme disease. *Clinical Infectious Diseases* 2015; 61: 248-250.
32. Bannwarth A. Chronic lymphocytic meningitis, inflammatory polyneuritis and 'rheumatism'. A contribution to the problem of 'allergy and nervous system' in two parts. *Archive für Psychiatrie und Nervenkrankheiten* 1941; 113: 284–376.
33. Barthold SW, Hodzic E, Imai DM et al. Ineffectiveness of tigecycline against persistent *Borrelia burgdorferi. Antimicrobial Agents Chemotherapy* 2010; 54: 643–651.
34. Bennet R, Lindgren V, Zweygberg-Wirgart B. *Borrelia* antibodies in children evaluated for Lyme neuroborreliosis. *Infection* 2008; 36(5): 463–466.
35. Berende A, Hofstede HJ, Vos FJ, Middendorp H van, Vogelaar ML, Tromp M, et al. Randomized trial of longer-term therapy for symptoms attributed to Lyme disease. *New England Journal of Medicine* 2016; 374: 1209–1220.
36. Berger BW. Dermatologic manifestations of Lyme disease. *Review Infectious Disease* 1989; 11(suppl. 6): S1475–S1481.
37. Biscardi S, Lorrot M, Marc E, Moulin F, Boutonnat-Faucher B, Heilbronner C, et al. *Mycoplasma pneumoniae* and asthma in children. *Clinical Infectious Diseases* 2004; 38: 1341-1346.

38. Blanc F, Jaulhac B, Fleury M, Sèze J de, Martino SJ de, Rémy V, Blaison G, Hansmann Y, Christmann D, Tranchant C. Relevance of the antibody index to diagnose Lyme neuroborreliosis among seropositive patients. *Neurology* 2007; 69(10): 953–958.
39. Bleati L, Péter O, Burgdorfer W, Aeschlimann A, Raoult D. Confirmation that *Rickettsia helvetica* sp. nov. is a distinct species of the spotted fever group of *Rickettsiae. International Journal of Systematic and Evolutionary Microbiology.* 1993; 43(3): 521–526. doi; 10.1099/00207713-43-3-521
40. Branda JA, Rosenberg ES. *Borrelia miyamotoi:* A lesson in disease discovery. *Annals Internal Medicine* 2013; 159(1): 61–62.
41. Bransfield RC. The psychoimmunology of Lyme/tick-borne diseases and its association with neuropsychiatric symptoms. *Open Neurology Journal* 2012; 6(suppl. 1–M3): 88–93.
42. Brorson O, Brorson SH. Transformation of cystic forms of *Borrelia burgdorferi* to normal, mobile spirochetes. *Infection* 1997; 25(4): 240–246.
43. Brorson O, Brorson SH. In vitro conversion of *Borrelia burgdorferi* to cystic forms in spinal fluid, and transformation to mobile spirochetes by incubation in BSK-H medium. *Infection* 1998; 26(3): 144–150.
44. Brorson O, Brorson SH. A rapid method for generating cystic forms of *Borrelia burgdorferi*, and their reversal to mobile spirochetes. *APMIS* 1998; 106(12): 1131–1141.
45. Brorson O, Brorson SH. An in vitro study of the susceptibility of mobile and cystic forms of *Borrelia burgdorferi* to metronidazole. *APMIS* 1999; 107(6): 566–576.
46. Brorson O, Brorson SH, Henriksen TH, Skogen PR, Schoyen R. Association between multiple sclerosis and cystic structures in cerebrospinal fluid. *Infection* 2001; 29(6): 315–319.
47. Brorson O, Brorson SH. Susceptibility of motile and cystic forms of *Borrelia burgdorferi* to ranitidine bismuth citrate. *International Microbiology* 2001; 4(4): 209–215.
48. Brorson O, Brorson SH. An in vitro study of the susceptibility of mobile and cystic forms of *Borrelia burgdorferi* to hydroxychloroquine. *International Microbiology* 2002; 5(1): 25–31.
49. Brorson O, Brorson SH. Grapefruit seed extract is a powerful in vitro agent against motile and cystic forms of *Borrelia burgdorferi sensu lato. Infection* 2007; 35(3): 206–208.

50. Brorson O, Brorson SH, Scythes J, MacAllister J, Wier A, Margulis L. Destruction of spirochete *Borrelia burgdorferi* round-body propagules (RBs) by the antibiotic tigecycline. *Proceedings National Academy Science USA* 2009; 106(44): 18656–18661.
51. Brunner M. Report refuting value of immune complexes to diagnose Lyme disease is invalid. *Clinical Vaccine Immunology* 2006; 13(2): 304–306.
52. Buchwald A. A case of diffuse idiopathic skin atrophy. *Archive of Dermatology and Syphilis* 1883; 10: 553–556.
53. Burckhardt JL. On the question of follicles and nucleation centres in the skin. *Frankfurt Journal of Pathology* 1911; 6(216): 1317–1319.
54. Burgdorfer W. On the occult infection in relapsing fevers. *Bulletin Society Pathology Exotic Filiales* 1954; 47(5): 664–667.
55. Burgdorfer W, Barbour AG, Hayes SF, Benach JL, Grunwaldt E, Davis JP. Lyme disease-a tick-borne spirochetosis? *Science* 1982; 216(4552): 1317–1319.
56. Buzzard EF. Spirochetes in MS (multiple sclerosis). *Lancet* 1911: 11(98).
57. Cairns V, Godwin J. Post-Lyme borreliosis syndrome: a meta-analysis of reported symptoms. *International Journal Epidemiology* 2005; 34: 1340–1345.
58. Cameron DJ, Johnson LB, Maloney EL. Evidence assessments and guideline recommendations in Lyme disease: the clinical management of known tick bites, erythema migrans rashes and persistent disease. *Expert Review Anti-infectious Therapy* 2014; 12(9): 1103–1135.
58a. Castelnuovo AD, Costanzo S, Antinori A, Berselli N, et al. Use of hydroxychloroquine in hospitalised COVID-19 patients is associated with reduced mortality: Findings from the observational multicentre Italian CORIST study. *Eur J Intern Med* 2020: 25 August (in press). doi:10.1016/j.ejim.2020.08.019
58b. Catteau L, Dauby N, Montourcy M, Bottieau E, et al. Low-dose Hydroxychloroquine Therapy and Mortality in Hospitalized Patients with COVID-19: A Nationwide Observational Study of 8075 Participants. *Int J Antimicrob Agents* 2020: 56(4): 106144. doi:10.1016/j.ijantimicag.2020.106144
59. Chmielewska-Badora J, Cisak E, Wojcik-Fatla A, Zwolinski J, Buczek A, Dutkiewicz J. Correlation of tests for detection of *Borrelia burgdorferi* sensu lato infection in patients with diagnosed

borreliosis. *Annals Agricultural Environmental Medicine* 2006; 13(2): 307–311.

60. Clark KL, Leydet B, Hartman S. Lyme borreliosis in human patients in Florida and Georgia, USA. *International of Journal Medical Science* 2013; 10(7): 915–931.
61. Cook MJ, Puri BK. Commercial test kits for detection of Lyme borreliosis: a meta-analysis of test accuracy. *International Journal of General Medicine* 2016; 18(9): 427–440.
62. Coyle PK. *Borrelia burgdorferi* antibodies in multiple sclerosis patients. *Neurology* 1989; 39(6): 760–761.
63. Crowle AJ, May MH. Inhibition of tubercle bacilli in cultured human macrophages by chloroquine used alone and in combination with streptomycin, isoniazid, pyrazinamide, and two metabolites of vitamin D. *Antimicrobial Agents Chemotherapy* 1990; 34(11): 2217–2222.
64. Danon SJ, Lee A. Other gastric helicobacters and spiral organisms. In: Mobley HLT, Mendz GL, Hazell SL (editors). *Helicobacter pylori*: Physiology and Genetics. ASM Press, Washington DC. 2001

64a. Davido B, Boussaid G, Vaugier I, Lansaman t, et al. Impact of medical care including anti-infective agents use on the prognosis of COVID-19 hospitalized patients over time. *Int J Antimicrob Agents* 2020: 56(4): 106129. doi:10.1016/j.ijantimicag.2020.106129

65. Davis GE, Burgdorfer W. On the susceptibility of the guinea pig to the relapsing fever spirochete *Borrelia duttonii. Bulletin Society Pathology Exotic Filiales* 1954; 47(4): 498–551.
66. de Koning J, Hoogkamp-Korstanje JA, Van der Linde MR, Crijns HJ. Demonstration of spirochetes in cardiac biopsies of patients with Lyme disease. *Journal of Infectious Disease* 1989; 160(1): 150–153.
67. Delchier J-C. Le lymphome gasrique du MALT, une infection maligne potentiel-lement curable – l'éradication d'*Helicobacter pylori. Gastroentérologie Clinique Biologique* 2003; 27(3–C2): 453–458.
68. de Long AK, Blossom B, Maloney EL, Phillips SE. Antibiotic retreatment of Lyme disease in patients with persistent symptoms: A biostatistical review of randomized, placebo-controlled, clinical trials. *Contemporary Clinical Trials* 2012; 33 (6): 1132–1142.

68a. de Truchis P, Assoumou L, Landman R, Mathez D, et al. Four-days-a-week antiretroviral maintenance therapy in virologically controlled HIV-1-infected adults: the ANRS 162-4D trial. *Antimicrob Chemother* 2018: 73(3): 738-747. doi: 10.1093/jac/dkx434.

69. Dietrich T, Geissdörfer W, Schlötzer-Schrehardt U, Holbach L, Schoerner C, Seitz B. *Borreli*a-associated crystalline keratopathy with intracorneal detection of *Borrelia garinii* by electron microscopy and polymerase chain reaction. *Cornea* 2008; 27(4): 498–500.

70. Donta ST. Tetracycline therapy for chronic Lyme disease. *Clinical Infectious Disease* 1997; 25(suppl 1): S52–S66.

71. Donta ST. Macrolide therapy of chronic Lyme disease. *Medical Science Monit*or 2003; 9(11): 136–142.

72. Donta ST, Noto RB, Vento JA. SPECT brain imaging in chronic Lyme disease. *Clinical Nuclear Medicine* 2012; 37(9): e219–222.

73. Dorward DW, Fischer ER, Brooks DM. Invasion and cytopathic killing of human lymphocytes by spirochetes causing Lyme disease. *Clinical Infectious Disease* 1997; 25(suppl 1): S2–S8.

74. Eldin C, Jaulhac B, Mediannikov JP, Raoult D. Values of diagnostic tests for the various species of spirochetes. *Médecine et Maladies Infectieuses* 2019; 49: 102–111. doi: 10.1016/j.medmal.2019.01.009.

75. Elsner RA, Hastey CJ, Olsen KJ, Baumgarth N. Suppression of long-lived humoral immunity following *Borrelia burgdorferi* infection. *PLoS Path*ogens 2015; 11(7): e1004976.

76. Embers ME, Ramamoorthy R, Philipp MT. Survival strategies of *Borrelia burgdorferi*, the aetiologic agent of Lyme disease. *Microbes Infections* 2004: 6: 312–318.

77. Embers ME, Barthold SW, Borda JT, Bowers L, Doyle L, Hodzic E et al. Persistence of *Borrelia burgdorferi* in Rhesus macaques following antibiotic treatment of disseminated infection. *PLoS ONE* 2012; 7(1): e29914. Erratum: *PLoS ONE* 2012; 7(4): 10.1371.

78. Embers ME et al. Variable manifestations, diverse seroreactivity and post-treatment persistence in non-human primates exposed to *Borrelia burgdorferi* by tick feeding. *PLoS ONE* 2017; 12. doi: 10.1371/journal.pone.0189071.

79. Eikeland R, Mygland A, Herlofson K, Ljostad U. European neuroborreliosis: quality of life 30 months after treatment. *Acta Neurology Scandinavia* 2011; 124: 349–354.

80. Fallon BA, Keilp JG, Cordera KM, Petkova E, Britton CB, Dwyer E et al. A randomized, placebo-controlled trial of repeated IV antibiotic therapy for Lyme encephalopathy. *Neurology* 2008; 70(13): 992–1003.
81. Fallon BA, Lipkin RB, Corbera KM, Yu S, Nobler MS, Keilp JG, Petkova E, Lisanby SH, Moeller JR, Slavov I, Van Heertum R, Mensh BD, Sackeim HA. Regional cerebral blood flow and metabolic rate in persistent Lyme encephalopathy. *Archives General Psychiatry* 2009; 66(5): 554–563.
82. Fehr JS, Bloemberg GV, Ritter C, Hombach M, Lüscher TF, Weber R, Keller PM. Septicemia caused by tick-borne bacterial pathogen *Candidatus* Neoehrlichia mikurensis. *Emerging Infectious Diseases* 2010; 16(7): 1127–1129.
83. Feller M, Huwiler K, Schoepfer A, Shang A, Furrer H, Egger M. Long-term antibiotic treatment for Crohn's disease: Systematic review and meta-analysis of placebo-controlled trials. *Clinical Infectious Diseases* 2010; 50(4): 473–478.
84. Feng J, Wang T, Shi W, Zhang S, Sullivan D, Auwaerter PG et al. Identification of novel activity against *Borrelia burgdorferi* persisters using an FDA approved drug library. *Emerging Microbes Infections* 2014; 3(7): e49.
85. Feng J, Auwaerter PG, Zhang Y. Drug combinations against *Borrelia burgdorferi* persisters in vitro: Eradication achieved by using daptomycin, cefoperazone and doxycycline. *PLoS ONE* 2015; 10(3): e0117207.
86. Feng J, Shi W, Zhang S, Zhang Y. Identification of new compounds with high activity against stationary phase *Borrelia burgdorferi* from the NCI compound collection. *Emerging Microbes Infections* 2015; 4(5): e31.
87. Feng J, Weitner M, Shi W, Zhang S, Sullivan D, Zhang Y. Identification of additional anti-persister activity against *Borrelia burgdorferi* from an FDA drug library. *Antibiotics* 2015; 4(3): 397–410.
88. Feng J, Shi W, Zhang S, Zhang Y. Persister mechanisms in *Borrelia burgdorferi*: Implications for improved intervention. *Emerging Microbes Infections* 2015; 4(8): e51.
89. Feng J, Shi W, Zhang S, Sullivan D, Auwaerter PG, Zhang Y. A drug combination screen identifies drugs active against amoxicillin-induced round bodies of in vitro *Borrelia burgdorferi* persisters

from an FDA drug library. *Frontiers in Microbiology* 2016; 7(743). doi:10.3389/fmicb.2016.00743.
90. Feng J, Shi W, Miklossy J, Tauxe GM, McMeniman CJ, Y Zhang. Identification of essential oils with strong activity against stationary phase of *Borrelia burgdorferi*. *Antibiotics* 2018; 7: 89.
91. Ferguson J. Cure unwanted? Exploring the chronic Lyme disease controversy and why conflicts of interest in practice guidelines may be guidelines guiding us down the wrong path. *American Journal Law Medicine* 2012; 38(1): 196–224.
92. Figoni J, Chirouze C, Hansmann Y, et al. Lyme borreliosis and other tick-borne diseases. Guidelines from the French scientific societies (I): Prevention, epidemiology, diagnosis. *Médecine et Maladies Infectieuses* 2019; 49: 318-334.
93. Fournier L, Roussel V, Couturier E, Jaulhac B, Goronflot T, Septfons A, De Martino S, Guerreiro S, Launay T, De Valk H *et al.* Epidémiologie de la Borréliose de Lyme en médecine générale, France Métropolitaine, 2009-2016. *Bull Epidemiol Hebdom* 2018; 19-20: 6.
94. Gao S, Li S, Ma Z, Liang S, Shan T, Zhang M, Zhu X, Zhang P, Liu G, Zhou F, Yuan X, Jia R, Potempa J, Scott DA, Lamont RJ, Wang H, Feng X. Presence of *Porphyromonas gingivalis* in esophagus and its association with the clinicopathological characteristics and survival in patients with esophageal cancer. *Infectious Agents Cancer* 2016; 11(3). doi:10.1186/s13027-016-0049-x.
95. Garg K, Meriläinen L et al. Evaluating polymicrobial immune responses in patients suffering from tick-borne diseases. *Nature Scientific Reports* 2018; 8: 15932.
96. Garin C, Bujadoux D. Paralysie par les tiques. *Journal des Maladies Régnantes à Lyon* 1922; 77: 765–767.
97. Gherardi RK, Coquet M, Chérin P, Authier FJ, Laforêt P, Bélec L et al. Macrophagic myofasciitis: An emerging entity. Groupe d'études et recherche sur les maladies musculaires acquises et dysimmunitaires (GERMMAd) de l'Association Française Contre les Myopathies (AFM). *Lancet* 1998; 352(9125): 347–352.
98. Gilden D et al. Prevalence and distribution of VZV in temporal arteries of patients with giant cell arteritis. *Neurology* 2015; 84(19): 1948–1955.

99. Girschick HJ, Huppertz HI, Rüssmann H, Krenn V, Karch H. Intracellular persistence of *Borrelia burgdorferi* in human synovial cells. *Rheumatology International* 1996; 16(3): 125–132.
100. Glaser V. Investigator profile: interview with Willy Burgdorfer, PhD. *Vector-Borne Zoonotic Disease* 2006: 6(4): 430–433.
101. Gompels LL, Smith A, Charles PJ, Rogers W, Soon-Shiong J, Mitchell A, et al. Single-blind randomized trial of combination antibiotic therapy in rheumatoid arthritis. *Journal of Rheumatology* 2006; 33(2): 224–227.
102. Grankvist A, Andersson PO, Mattsson M, Sender M, Vaht K, Höper L et al. Infections with the tick-borne bacterium '*Candidatus* Neoehrlichia mikurensis' mimic non-infectious conditions in patients with B cell malignancies or auto-immune diseases. *Clinical Infectious Diseases* 2014; 58(12): 1716–1722.
103. Greenstein RJ. Is Crohn's disease caused by a mycobacterium? Comparisons with leprosy, tuberculosis and Johne's disease. *Lancet Infectious Diseases* 2003; 3(8): 507–514.
104. Gui GP, Thomas PR, Tzard ML, Lake J, Sanderson JD, Hermon-Taylor J. Two-year-outcomes analysis of Crohn's disease treated with rifabutin and macrolide antibiotics. *Journal Antimicrobial Chemotherapy* 1997; 39(3): 393–400.
105. Guyatt GH, Oxman AD, Vist GE et al. GRADE: an emerging consensus on rating quality of evidence and strength of recommendations. *BMJ* 2008; 336: 924–926.
106. Haddad E et al. Holistic approach in patients with presumed Lyme borreliosis leads to less than 10% of confirmation and more than 80% antibiotic failure. *Clinical Infectious Diseases* 2018. doi.org/10.1093/cid/ciy799.
107. Hao Q, Hou X, Geng Z, Wan K. Distribution of *Borrelia burgdorferi sensu lato* in China. *Journal of Clinical Microbiology* 2011; 49(2): 647–650.
108. Harvey WT, Martz D. Motor neuron disease recovery associated with IV ceftriaxone and anti-*Babesia* therapy. *Acta Neurologica Scandinavia* 2006; 115(2): 129–131.
109. Haupl T, Hahn G, Rittig M et al. Persistence of *Borrelia burgdorferi* in ligamentous tissue from a patient with chronic Lyme borreliosis. *Arthritis Rheumatology* 1993; 36: 1621–1626.

110. Herxheimer K, Hartmann K. Ueber Acrodermatitis chronica atrophicans. *Archive für Dermatologie und Syphilis* 1902; 61(1): 57–76.
111. Hodzic E, Feng S, Holden K, Freet KJ, Barthold SW. Persistence of *Borrelia burgdorferi* following antibiotic treatment in mice. *Antimicrobial Agents Chemotherapy* 2008; 52(5): 1728–1736.
112. Hokynar K et al. *Chlamydia*-like organisms (CLO) in Finnish *Ixodes ricinus* and human skin. *Microorganisms* 2016. doi: 10.3390/microorganisms4030028.
113. Holl-Wieden A, Suerbaum S, Girschick HJ. Seronegative Lyme arthritis. *Rheumatology International* 2007; 27(11): 1091–1093.
114. Horowitz R, Freeman P. The use of dapsone as a novel 'persister' drug in the treatment of chronic Lyme disease/post treatment Lyme disease syndrome. *Journal Clinical Experimental Dermatological Research* 2016; 7(3). doi:10.4172/2155-9554.1000345.
115. Horowitz RI, Freeman PR. Are mycobacterium drugs effective for treatment resistant Lyme disease, tick-borne co-infections, and autoimmune disease? *JSM Arthritis* 2016; 1(2): 1008.
116. Hunfeld KP, Ruzic-Sabljic E, Norris DE, Kraiczy P, Strl F. In vitro susceptibility testing of *Borrelia burgdorferi* sensu lato isolates cultured from patients with erythema migrans before and after antimicrobial chemotherapy. *Antimicrobial Agents Chemotherapy* 2005; 49(4): 1294–1301.
117. Jaulhac B, Saunier A, Caumes E, et al. Lyme borreliosis and other tick-borne diseases. Guidelines from the French scientific societies (II): Biological diagnosis, treatment, persistent symptoms after documented or suspected Lyme borreliosis. *Médecine et Maladies Infectieuses* 2019; 49: 335-346.
118. Johnson L, Sticker R. Attorney General forces Infectious Diseases Society of America to redo Lyme guidelines due to flawed development process. *Journal of Medical Ethics* 2009: 35; 283-288. dx.doi.org/10.1136/jme.2008.026526
119. Karan L, Makenov M, Kolyasnikova N, Stukolova M, Toporkova M, Olenkova O. Dynamics of spirochetemia and early PCR detection of *Borrelia miyamotoi. Emerg Infect Dis* 2018. 24; 860-867.
120. Keller A, Graefen A, Ball M, Matzas M, Boisguerin V, Maixner F, Leidinger P, Backes C et al. New insights into the Tyrolean Iceman's origin and phenotype as inferred by whole-genome

sequencing. *Nature Communications* 2012; 3(698). doi:10.1038/ncomms1701.

121. Kennedy AG. Differential diagnosis and the suspension of judgment. *Journal Medical Philosophy* 2013; 38(5): 487–500.

122. Klempner MS, Hu LT, Evans J, Schmid CH, Johnson GM, Trevino RP, Norton D, Levy L, Wall D, McCall J, Kosinski M, Weinstein A. Two controlled trials of antibiotic treatment in patients with persistent symptoms and a history of Lyme disease. *New England Journal Medicine* 2001; 345: 85–92.

123. Krupp LB, Hyman LG, Grimson R, Coyle PK, Melville P, Ahnn S et al. Study and treatment of post-Lyme disease (STOP-LD): A randomized double masked clinical trial. *Neurology* 2003; 60(12): 1923–1930.

124. Kugeler KJ, Farley GM, Forrester JD, Mead PS. Geographic distribution and expansion of human Lyme disease, United States. *Emerging Infectious Diseases* 2015: 21(8): 1455–1457.

124a. Lagier J-C, Million M, Gautret P, Colson P, Cortaredona S, Giraud-Gatineau A, et al. Outcomes of 3,737 COVID-19 patients treated with hydroxychloroquine/azithromycin and other regimens in Marseille, France: A retrospective analysis. *Travel Med Infectious Dis* 2020; 36: 101791. doi.org/10.1016/j.tmaid.2020.101791.

125. Lamb R, Ozsvari B, Lisanti CL, Tanowitz HB, Howell A, Martinez-Outschoorn UE et al. Antibiotics that target mitochondria effectively eradicate cancer stem cells, across multiple tumor types: treating cancer like an infectious disease. *Oncotarget* 2015; 6(7): 4569–4584.

126. Lantos PM, Charini WA, Medoff G, Moro MH, Muschatt DM, Parsonnet J et al. Final report of the Lyme disease review panel of the Infectious diseases Society of America. *Clinical Infectious Diseases* 2010; 51(1): 1–5.

127. Lawrence C, Lipton RB, Lowy FD, Coyle PK. Seronegative chronic relapsing neuroborreliosis. *European Neurology* 1995; 35: 113–117.

128. Lecuit M, Abachin E, Martin A, Poyard C et al. Immunoproliferative small intestinal disease associated with *Campylobacter jejuni*. *New England Journal Medicine* 2004; 350: 239–248.

129. Lee DJ, Vielmeyer O. Analysis of overall level of evidence behind Infectious diseases Society of America practice guidelines. *Archives International Medicine* 2011: 171(1): 18–22.
130. Lee SH, Vigliotti JS, Vigliotti VS, Jones W, Shearer DM. Detection of *Borreliae* in archived sera from patients with clinically suspect Lyme disease. *International Journal of Molecular Science* 2014; 15(3): 4284–4298.
131. Lee-Lewandrowski E, Chen Z, Branda J, Baron J, Kaufman HW. Laboratory Blood-Based Testing for Lyme Disease at a National Reference Laboratory. *Am J Clin Pathol* 2019: 152: 6.
132. Leibovitch EC, Jacobson S. Evidence linking HHV-6 with multiple sclerosis: An update. *Current Opinion in Virology* 2014; 9, 127-133.
133. Lewis K. Persister cells, dormancy and infectious disease. *Nature Reviews Microbiology* 2007; 5(1): 48–56.
134. Lipschütz B. About a rare form of erythema (erythema chronicum migrans). *Archive of Dermatology and Syphilis* 1913; 118(1): 349–356.
135. Liu F, Guo X, Wu R, Ou J, Zheng Y, Zhang B et al. Minocycline supplementation for treatment of negative symptoms in early-phase schizophrenia: A double blind, randomized, controlled trial. *Schizophrenia Research* 2014; 153(1-3): 169–170.
136. Livengood JA, Gilmore RD Jr. Invasion of human neuronal and glial cells by an infectious strain of *Borrelia burgdorferi*. *Microbes Infections* 2006; 8(14–15): 2832–2840.
137. Lopes de Carvalho I, Fonseca JE, Brands JG, Ullmann A, Hojgaard A, Zeidner N, Nuncio MS. Vasculitis-like syndrome associated with *Borrelia lusitaniae* infection. *Clinical Rheumatology* 2008; 27(12): 1587–1591.
138. Lubke LL, Garon CF. The antimicrobial agent melittin exhibits powerful in vitro inhibitory effects on the Lyme disease spirochete. *Clinical Infectious Disease* 1997; 25(suppl. 1): S48–S51.
139. MacDonald AB. Concurrent neocortical borreliosis and Alzheimer's disease: demonstration of a spirochetal cyst form. *Annals NY Academy Science* 1988; 539: 468–470.
140. MacDonald AB. Spirochetal cyst forms in neurodegenerative disorders, … hiding in plain sight. *Medical Hypotheses* 2006; 67(4): 819–832.

140a. Maizels RM. Parasitic helminth infections and the control of human allergic and autoimmune disorders. *Clinical Microbiology and Infection* 2016; 22(6): 481–486. doi: 10-1016/j.cmi.2016.04.024

141. Makhani N, Morris SK, Page AV, Brophy J, Lindsay LR, Banwell BL, Richardson SE. A twist on Lyme: the challenge of diagnosing European Lyme neuroborreliosis. *Journal Clinical Microbiology* 2011; 49(1): 455–457.

142. Mantovani E, Costa IP, Gauditano G, Bonoldi VL, Higuchi ML, Yoshinari NH. Description of Lyme disease-like syndrome in Brazil. Is it a new tick-borne disease or Lyme disease variation? *Brazilian Journal Medical Biological Research* 2007; 40(4): 443–456.

143. Marangoni A, Sparacino M, Cavrini F, Storni E, Mondardini V, Sambri V, Cevenini R. Comparative evaluation of three different ELISA methods for the diagnosis of early culture-confirmed Lyme disease in Italy. *Journal Medical Microbiology* 2005; 54(Pt 4): 361–367.

144. Margos G, Piesman J, Lane RS, Ogden NH, Sing A, Straubinger RK, Fingerle V. *Borrelia kurtenbachii* sp. nov., a widely distributed member of the *Borrelia burgdorferi sensu lato* species complex in North America. *International Journal Systematic Evolutionary Microbiology* 2014; 64(Pt 1): 128–130.

145. Masters E, Lynxwiler P, Rawlings J. Spirochetemia after continuous high-dose oral amoxicillin therapy. *Infectious Disease Clinical Practice* 1994; 3(3): 207–208.

145a. Mathez D, de Truchis P, Ledu D, Melchior JC, et al. Four days a week or less on appropriate anti-HIV drug combinations provided long-term optimal maintenance in 94 patients: the ICCARRE project. *FASEB Journal* 2015: 29(6) : 2223-2234. doi.org/10.1096/fj.14-260315

146. Mavin S, Milner RM, Evans R, Chatterton JM, Joss AW, Ho-Yen DO. The use of local isolates in Western blots improves serological diagnosis of Lyme disease in Scotland. *Journal of Medical Microbiology* 2007; 56(Pt 1): 47–51.

147. Mavin S. Evans R. Milner RM. Chatterton JM, Ho-Yen DO. Local *Borrelia burgdorferi sensu stricto* and *Borrelia afzelii* strains in a single mixed antigen improves Western blot sensitivity. *Journal Clinical Pathology* 2009; 62(6): 552–554.

148. Mechelli R, Manzari C, Policano C, Annese A, Picardi E, Umeton R, et al. Epstein-Barr virus genetic variants are associated with multiple sclerosis. *Neurology* 2015; 31(84): 1362–1368.
149. Mediannikov O, Socolovschi C, Bassene H, Diatta G, Ratmanov P, Fenollar F, et al. *Borrelia crocidurae* infection in acutely febrile patients, Senegal. *Emerging Infectious Diseases* 2014; 20: 1335-1338.
150. Meijer AC, Stijnen T, Wasser MN, Hamming JP, Bockel JH van, Lindeman JH. Doxycycline for stabilization of abdominal aortic aneurysms: A randomized trial. *Annals of Internal Medicine* 2013; 159(12): 815–823.
151. Melaun C, Zotzmann S, Santaella VG, Werblow A, Zumkowski-Xylander H, Kraiczy P et al. Occurrence of *Borrelia burgdorferi* s.l. in different genera of mosquitoes (*Culicidae*) in Central Europe. *Ticks Tick Borne Disease* 2016; 7(2): 256–263.
152. Melia MT, Auwaerter P. Time for a different approach to Lyme disease and long-term symptoms. *New England Journal of Medicine* 2016; 374(13): 1277–1278.
153. Meriläinen L, Herranen A, Schwarzbach A, Gilbert L. Morphological and biochemical features of *Borrelia burgdorferi* pleomorphic forms. *Microbiology* 2015; 161(Pt 1): 516–527.
154. Meriläinen L, Brander H, Herranen A, Schwarzbach A, Gilbert L. Pleomorphic forms of *Borrelia burgdorferi* induce distinct immune responses. *Microbes Infection* 2016; 18(7–8): 484–495.
155. Middelveen MJ, Burke J, Sapi E, Bandoski C, Filusch KR, Wang Y et al. Culture and identification of *Borrelia* spirochetes in human vaginal and seminal secretions. *F1000Research* 2014; 3(309). doi:10.12688/f1000research.5778.3.
156. Middleveen MJ, Sapi E, et al. Persistent *Borrelia* infection in patients with ongoing symptoms of Lyme disease. *Healthcare* 2018; 6(2): 33. doi: 10.3390/healthcare6020033.
157. Miklossy J. Alzheimer's disease – a neurospirochetosis. Analysis of the evidence fol- lowing Koch's and Hill's criteria. *Journal of Neuroinflammation* 2011; 8: 90.
158. Miklossy J. Chronic or late Lyme neuroborreliosis: Analysis of evidence compared to chronic or late neurosyphilis. *Open Neurology Journal* 2012; 6: 146–157.
159. Miklossy J. Historic evidence to support a causal relationship between spirochetal infections and Alzheimer's disease. *Frontiers Aging Neuroscience* 2015; 7. doi:10.3389/ fnagi.2015.00046.

160. Moore A, Nelson C, Molins C, et al. Common clinical pitfalls and future directions for laboratory diagnosis of Lyme disease, United States. *Emerging Infectious Diseases* 2016; 22: 1169-1177.
161. Moutailler S, Valiente-Moro C, Vaumourin E, Michelet L, Tran FH, Devilliers E, et al. Co-infection of ticks; The rule rather than the exception. *PLoS Neglected Tropical Diseases* 2016; 10(3): e0004539.
162. Muller I, Freitag MH, Poggensee G, Scharnetzky E, Straube E, Schoerner C, Hlobil H, Hagedorn HJ, Stanek G, Schubert-Unkmeir A, *et al*. Evaluating frequency, diagnostic quality, and cost of Lyme borreliosis testing in Germany: a retrospective model analysis. *Clin Dev Immunol* 2012, 2012: 595427.
163. Murgia R, Cinco M. Induction of cystic forms by different stress conditions in *Borrelia burgdorferi*. *APMIS* 2004; 112(1): 57–62.
164. Nanagara R, Duray PH, Schumacher HR Jr. Ultrastructural demonstration of spirochetal antigens in synovial fluid and synovial membrane in chronic Lyme disease: Possible factors contributing to persistence in organisms. *Human Pathology* 1996; 27(10): 1025–1034.
165. Nields JA, Kveton J.F. Tullio phenomenon and seronegative Lyme borreliosis. *Lancet* 1991; 338(8759): 128–129.
166. Noah DL, Ostroff SM, Cropper TL, Thacker SB. US military officer participation in the Centers for Disease Control and Prevention's Epidemic Intelligence Service (1951–2001). *Military Medicine* 2003; 168(5): 368–372.
167. Nordstrand A, Bunikis I, Larsson C, Tsogbe K, Schwan TG, Nilsson M, et al. Tick-borne relapsing fever diagnosis obscured by malaria, Togo. *Emerging Infectious Diseases* 2007. doi: 10.3201/eid1301.060670.
168. O'Dell JR, Elliott JR, Mallek JA, Mikuls TR, Weaver CA, Glickstein S, et al. Treatment of early seropositive rheumatoid arthritis. Doxycycline plus methotrexate versus methotrexate alone. *Arthritis Rheumatology* 2006; 54(2): 621–627.
169. O'Dell JR, Blakely KW, Mallek JA, Eckhoff PJ, Leff RD, Wees SJ et al. Treatment of early seropositive rheumatoid arthritis. A two-year, double-blind comparison of minocycline and hydroxychloroquine. *Arthritis Rheumatolgy* 2001; 44(10): 2235–2241.
170. Ogden NH, Margos G, Aanensen DM, Drebot MA, Feil EJ, Hanincova K, Tyler S, Lindsay LR. Investigation of genotypes

of *Borrelia burgdorferi* in *Ixodes scapularis* ticks collected during surveillance in Canada. *Applied Environmental Microbiology* 2011; 77(10): 3244–3254.

171. Ogrendik M. Effects of clarithromycin in patients with active rheumatoid arthritis. *Current Medical Research and Opinion* 2007; 23(3): 515–522.
172. Oksi J, Nikoskelainen J, Viljanen MK. Comparison of oral cefixime and intravenous ceftriaxone followed by oral amoxicillin in disseminated Lyme borreliosis. *European Journal Clinical Microbiology Infectious Disease* 1998; 17: 715–719.
173. Oksi J, Marjamäki M, Nikoskelainen, Viljanen MK. *Borrelia burgdorferi* detected by culture and PCR in clinical relapse of disseminated Lyme borreliosis. *Annals of Medicine* 1999; 31: 225–232.
174. Paules CI et al. Tickborne diseases – Confronting a growing threat. *New England Journal of Medicine* 2018. doi: 10.1056/NEJMp1807870.
175. Pedersen MG, Mortensen PB, Norgaard-Pedersen B, Postolache TT. *Toxoplasma gondii* infection and self-directed violence in mothers. *Archives of General Psychiatry* 2012; 69(11): 1123–1130.
176. Pfister HW, Preac-Mursic V, Wilske B et al. Randomised comparison of ceftriaxone and cefotaxime in Lyme neuroborreliosis. *Journal of Infectious Disease* 1991; 163: 311–318.
177. Phillips SE, Mattman LH, Hulinska D, Moayad H. A proposal for the reliable culture of *Borrelia burgdorferi* from patients with chronic Lyme disease, even from those previously aggressively treated. *Infection* 1998; 26(6): 364–367.
178. Pick PJ. On a new disease: erythromelie. *Negotiations of the Society of German Natural Scientists* 1894; 66(II): 336.
179. Pierer M, Rothe K, Quandt D, Schulz A, Rossol M, Scholz R et al. Association of anticytomegalovirus seropositivity with more severe joint destruction and more frequent joint surgery in rheumatoid arthritis. *Arthritis Rheumatology* 2012; 64: 1740–1749.
180. Portillo A, Santibanez P, Palomar AM, Santibanez S, Oteo JA. "*Candidatus* Neoehrlichia mikurensis" in Europe. *N Microbes N Infections* 2018; 22: 30-36.
181. Preac-Mursic V, Pfister HW, Spiegel et al. First isolation of *Borrelia burgdorferi* from an iris biopsy. *Journal of Clinical Neuroophthalmology* 1993; 13: 155–161.

182. Preac-Mursic V, Weber K, Pfister HW. Survival of *Borrelia burgdorferi* in antibiotically treated patients with Lyme borrreliosis. *Infection* 1989; 17: 355–359.
183. Preac-Mursic V, Pfister HW, Spiegel H, Burk R, Wilske B, Reinhardt S, et al. Formation and cultivation of *Borrelia burgdorferi* spheroplast-L-form variants. *Infection* 1996; 24(3): 218–226.
184. Priem S, Burmester GR, Kamradt T, Wolbart K, Rittig MG, Krause A. Detection of *Borrelia burgdorferi* by polymerase chain reaction in synovial membrane, but not in synovial fluid from patients with persisting Lyme arthritis after antibiotic therapy. *Annals Rheumatology Disease* 1998; 57(2): 118–121.
185. Pritt BS, Mead PS, Johnson DK, Neitzel DF, Respicio-Kingry LB, Davis JP et al. Identification of a novel pathogenic *Borrelia* species causing Lyme borreliosis with unusually high spirochaetemia: A descriptive study. *Lancet Infectious Diseases* 2016; 16(5): 556–564.
186. Raguet S, Le Strat Y, Chouin L, Hansmann Y, Martinot M, Kieffer P, De Martino S, Jaulhac B, Wendling MJ, Velay A *et al.* Incidence de la borréliose de Lyme dans les départements alsaciens, étude Alsa(ce)tique, 2014-2015. *Bull Epidemiol Hebdom* 2018; 19-20: 7.
187. Raoult D. Lack of knowledge can anger patients with chronic diseases. *Lancet Infectious Diseases* 2012; 12(9): 654–655.
188. Reik L Jr, Burgdorfer W, Donaldson JO. Neurologic abnormalities in Lyme disease without erythema chronicum migrans. *American Journal of Medicine* 1986; 81(1): 73–78.
189. Rizzoli A, Hauffe H., Carpi G, Vourc'h GI, Neteler M, Rosà R. Lyme borreliosis in Europe. *Eurosurveillance* 2011; 16(27): 1–8.
190. Rolain JM, Colson P, Raoult D. Recycling of chloroquine and its hydroxyl analogue to face bacterial, fungal and viral infections in the 21st century. *International Journal of Antimicrobial Agents* 2007; 30(4): 297–308.
191. Robinot R, Robinot E. Chronic *Borrelia burgdorferi* infection triggers NKT lymphomagenesis. *Blood* 2018; 132(25): 2691–2695. doi:10.1182/blood-2018-07-863381.
192. Rudenko N, Golovchenko M, Ruzek D, Piskunova N, Mallatova N, Grubhoffer L. Molecular detection of *Borrelia bissettii* DNA in serum samples from patients in the Czech

Republic with suspected borreliosis. *FEMS Microbiology Letter* 2009; 292(2): 274–281.

193. Rudenko N, Golovchenko M, Grubhoffer L, Oliver JH Jr. Updates on *Borrelia burgdorferi* sensu lato complex with respect to public health. *Ticks Tick-Borne Diseases* 2011: 2(3): 123–128.
194. Sackett DL, Rosenberg WM, Gray JA, Haynes RB, Richardson WS. Evidence based medicine: what it is and what it isn't. *BMJ* 1996; 312: 71–72. doi.org/10.1136/bmj.312.7023.71.
195. Sapi E, Balasubramanian K, Poruri A, Maghsoudlou JS, Socarras KM, Timmaraju AV et al. Evidence of in vivo existence of *Borrelia* biofilm in borrelial lymphocytomas. *European Journal of Microbiological Immunology* 2016; 6(1): 9–24.
196. Sapi E, Kasliwala RS, Ismail H, et al. The long-term persistence of *Borrelia burgdorferi* antigens and DNA in the tissues of a patient with Lyme disease. *Antibiotics* 2019; 183. doi: 10.3390/antibiotics8040183
197. Savarino A, Di Trani L, Donatelli I, Cauda R, Cassone A. New insights into the antiviral effects of chloroquine. et al. *Lancet Infectious Diseases* 2006. doi: 10.1016/S1473-3099(06)70361-9.
198. Schardt FW. Clinical effects of fluconazole in patients with neuroborreliosis. *European Journal Medical Research* 2004; 9(7): 334–336.
199. Scher JU, Sczesnak A, Longman RS, Segata N, Ubeda C, Bielski C et al. Expansion of intestinal *Prevotella copri* correlates with enhanced susceptibility to arthritis. *eLife* 2013; 2: e01202.
200. Schmidli J, Hunziker T, Moesli P, Schaad UB. Cultivation of *Borrelia burgdorferi* from joint fluid three months after treatment of facial palsy due to Lyme borreliosis. *Journal of Infectious Diseases* 1988; 158: 905–906.
201. Schouls LM, Van de Pol I, Rijpkema SG, Schot CS. Detection and identification of *Ehrlichia*, *Borrelia burgdorferi sensu lato*, and *Bartonella* species in Dutch *Ixodes ricinus* ticks. *Journal of Clinical Microbiology* 1999; 37(7): 2215–2222.
202. Schutzer SE, Coyle PK, Belman AL, Golightly MG, Drulle J. Sequestration of antibody to *Borrelia burgdorferi* in immune complexes in seronegative Lyme disease. *Lancet* 1990; 335(8685): 312–315.
203. Schutzer SE, Body BA, Boyle J, et al. Direct diagnostic tests for Lyme disease. *Clinical Infectious Diseases* 2019; 68: 1052-1057.

204. Schwan TG, Anderson JM, Lopez JE, Fischer RJ, Raffel SJ, McCoy BN, Safronetz D, Sogoba N, Maïga O, Traoré SF. Endemic foci of the tick-borne relapsing fever spirochete *Borrelia crocidurae* in Mali, West Africa, and the potential for human infection. *PLoS Neglected Tropical Diseases* 2012; 6(11): e1924.
205. Scott IA, Guyatt GH. Suggestions for improving guideline utility and trustworthiness. *Evidence Based Medicine* 2013; 19: 41–46.
206. Scrimenti RJ. Erythema chronicum migrans. *Archives in Dermatology* 1970; 102(1): 104–105.
207. Shadick NA, Phillips CB, Logigian EL et al. The long-term clinical outcomes of Lyme disease. A population-based retrospective cohort study. *Annals Internal Medicine* 1994; 121: 905–908.
208. Sharma B, Brown AV, Matluck NE, Hu LT, Lewis K. *Borrelia burgdorferi*, the causative agent of Lyme disease, forms drug-tolerant persister cells. *Antimicrobial Agents Chemotherapy* 2015; 59(8): 4616–4624.
209. Simon M, Pariente B, Lambert J, Cosnes J, Bouhnik Y, Marteau P, et al. Long-term outcomes of thalidomide therapy for adults with refractory Crohn's disease. *Clinical Gastroenterology Hepatology* 2016; 14(7): 966–972.
210. Skogman BH, Glimaker K, Nordwall M, et al. Long-term clinical outcome after Lyme neuroborreliosis in childhood. *Pediatrics* 2012; 130: 262–269.
211. Smith GC, Pell JP. Parachute use to prevent death and major trauma related to gravitational challenge: Systematic review of randomized controlled trials. *BMJ* 2003; 327(7429): 1459–1461.
212. Socarras KM, Theophilus PAS, Torres JP, Gupta K, Sapi E. Antimicrobial activity of bee venom and melittin against *Borrelia burgdorferi*. *Antibiotics* 2017; 6; 31. doi: 10.3390/antibiotics6040031.
213. Stanek G, Reiter M. The expanding Lyme *Borrelia* complex – clinical significance of genomic species? *Clinical Microbiology Infection* 2011; 17(4): 487–493.
214. Steere AC, Malawista SE, Hardin JA, Ruddy S, Askenase PW, Andiman WA. Erythema chronicum migrans and Lyme arthritis. The enlarging clinical spectrum. *Annals of Internal Medicine* 1977; 86(6): 685–698.
215. Steere AC, Malawista SE, Snydman DR, Shope RE, Andiman WA, Ross MR, Steele FM. Lyme arthritis : An epidemic

of oligoarticular arthritis in children and adults in three Connecticut communities. *Arthritis Rheumatology* 1977: 20(1): 7–17.

216. Steere AC, Grodzicki RL, Kornblatt AN, Craft JE, Barbour AG, Burgdorfer W, Schmid GP, Johnson E, Malawista SE. The spirochetal etiology of Lyme disease. *New England Journal of Medicine* 1983; 308(13): 733–740.
217. Straubinger RK, Summers BA, Chang YF, Appel MJ. Persistence of *Borrelia burgdorferi* in experimentally infected dogs after antibiotic treatment. *Journal of Clinical Microbiology* 1997; 35(1): 111–116.
218. Straubinger RK. PCR-based quantification of *Borrelia burgdorferi* organisms in canine tissues over a 500-day post-infection period. *Journal of Clinical Microbiology* 2000; 38(6): 2191–2199.
219. Stricker RB, Moore DH, Winger EE. Clinical and immunologic evidence for transmission of Lyme disease through intimate human contact. *Journal of Investigative Medicine* 2004; 52(suppl. 1): S151.
220. Stricker RB. Counterpoint: Long term antibiotic therapy improves persistent symptoms associated with Lyme disease. *Clinical Infectious Disease* 2007; 45(2): 149–157.
221. Stricker RB, Middleveen MJ. Sexual transmission of Lyme disease: Challenging the tickborne disease paradigm. *Expert Review Anti-Infectious Therapies* 2015; 13(1): 1303–1306.
222. Stricker RB, Johnson L. Lyme disease: Call for a 'Manhattan Project' to combat the epidemic. *PLoS Pathogen* 2014; 10(1): e1003796.
223. Strle F, Preac-Mursic V, Cimperman J, et al. Azithromycin vesus doxycycline for treatment of erythema migrans: clinical and microbiological findings. *Infection* 1993; 21: 83–88.
224. Strle F, Stanek G. Clinical manifestations of Lyme borreliosis. *Current Problems in Dermatology* 2009; 37: 51–110.
225. Sykes RA, Makiello P. An estimate of Lyme borreliosis incidence in Western Europe. *J Public Health* 2017; 39: 74-81. doi: 10.1093/pubmed/fdw017.
226. Tager FA, Fallon BA, Keilp J, Rissenberg M, Ray Jones C, Liebowitz MR. A controlled study of cognitive deficits in children with chronic Lyme disease. *Journal Neuropsychology Clinical Neurosciences* 2001; 13(4): 500–507.

227. Tan AH, Mahadeva S, Marras C, Thalha AM, Kiew CK, Yeat CM, et al. *Helicobacter pylori* infection is associated with worse severity of Parkinson's disease. *Parkinsonism Relationship Disorders* 2015; 21(3): 221–225.

228. Telford SR 3rd, Goethert HK, Molloy PJ, Berardi VP, Chowdri HR, Gugliotta JL et al. *Borrelia miyamotoi* disease: Neither Lyme disease nor relapsing fever. *Clinical Laboratory Medicine* 2015; 35(4): 867–882.

229. Tveitnes D, Oymar K, Natas O. Laboratory data in children with Lyme neuroborreliosis, relation to clinical presentation and duration of symptoms. *Scandinavian Journal of Infectious Disease* 2009; 41(5): 355–362.

230. Valesova M, Trnavsky K, Hulinska D, Alusik S, Janousek J, Jirous J. Detection of *Borrelia* in the synovial tissue from a patient with Lyme borreliosis by electron microscopy. *Journal of Rheumatology* 1989; 16(11): 1502–1505.

231. Varela AS, Luttrell MP, Howerth EW, Moore VA, Davidson WR, Stallknecht DE, Little SE. First culture isolation of *Borrelia lonestari,* putative agent of Southern tick-associated rash illness. *Journal of Clinical Microbiology* 2004; 42(3): 1163–1169.

232. Vayssier-Taussat M, Moutailler S, Michelet L, Devillers E, Bonnet S, Cheval J, Hébert C, Eloit M. Next generation sequencing uncovers unexpected bacterial pathogens in ticks in Western Europe. *PLoS ONE* 2013; 8(11): e81439.

233. Vayssier-Taussat M, Moutailler S, Féménia F, Raymond P, Croce O, La Scola B, et al. Identification of novel zoonotic activity of *Bartonella* spp. *Emerging Infectious Disease* 2016; 22(3): 457–462.

234. Vial L, Diatta G, Tall A, Ba EH, Bouganali H, Durand P, et al. Incidence of tick-borne relapsing fever in West Africa: longitudinal study. *Lancet* 2006; 368: 37-43.

235. Vincent MJ, Bergeron E, Benjannet S, et al. Chloroquine is a potent inhibitor of SARS coronavirus infection and spread. *Virology Journal* 2005; 2: 69.

236. Waisbren BA. The Emperor's New Clothes, Chronic Lyme disease, and the Infectious Disease Society of America. In: *Treatment of chronic Lyme disease: Fifty-one case reports and essays in their regard. Essay 4. The Lyme Handbook* 25 April 2011. https://lymehandbook.com/2011/04/251

237. Wallet F, Labalette P, Herwegh S, Loïez C, Margaron F, Courcol RJ. Molecular diagnosis of a bilateral panuveitis due to *Borrelia burgdorferi sensu lato* by cerebral spinal fluid analysis. *Journal Infectious Disease* 2008; 61(3): 214–215.
238. Weber K, Wilske B, Preac-Mursic V, Thurmayr R. Azithromycin versus penicillin V for the treatment of early Lyme borreliosis. *Infection* 1993; 21: 367–372.
239. Wojciechowska-Koszko I, Maczynska I, Szych Z, Giedrys-Kalemba S. Serodiagnosis of borreliosis: Indirect immunofluorescence assay, enzyme-linked immunosorbent assay and immunoblotting. *Archivum Immunologiae et Therapiae Experimentalis* 2011; 59(1): 69–77.
240. Wormser GP. Early Lyme disease. *New England Journal of Medicine* 2006; 354: 2794–2801.
241. Wormser GP, Dattwyler RJ, Shapiro ED, et al. The clinical assessment, treatment, and prevention of Lyme disease, human granulocytic anaplasmosis, and babesiosis: Clinical practice guidelines by the Infectious Diseases Society of America. *Clinical Infectious Diseases* 2006; 43(9): 1089–1134.
242. Wormser GP, Weizner E, McKenna D, Nadelman RB, Scavarda C, Molla I, et al. Long-term assessment of health-related quality of life in patients with culture-confirmed early Lyme disease. *Clinical Infectious Disease* 2015; 61(2): 244–247.
243. Wormser GP, Nadelman RB, Schwartz I. The amber theory of Lyme erthritis: initial description and clinical implications. *Clinical Rheumatology* 2012; 31: 989-994.
244. Yrjänäinen H, Hytönen J, Hartiala P, Oksi J, Viljanen MK. Persistence of borrelial DNA in the joints of *Borrelia burgdorferi*-infected mice after ceftriaxone treatment. *APMIS* 2010: 118(9): 665–673.
245. Zhang Y, Träskman-Bendz L, Janelidze S, Langeberg P, Saleh A, Constantine N. et al. *Toxoplasma gondii* immunoglobulin G antibodies and nonfatal suicidal self-directed violence. *Journal Clinical Psychiatry* 2012; 73(8): 1069–1076.
245. Zhang Y. Persisters, persistent infections and the yin–yang model. *Emerging Microbes Infections* 2014; 3: e3.
246. Ziska MH, Donta ST, Demarest FC. Physician preferences in the diagnosis and treatment of Lyme disease in the United States. *Infection* 1996; 24(2): 182–186.

General articles

247. Baumber N. Will G8 funding for dementia research recognise the involvement of stealth pathogens in the global pandemic? *The Pharmaceutical Journal* 15 September 2014.

248. Grann D. Stalking Dr Steere over Lyme disease. *The New York Times,* 17 June 2001.

Books

Albertat J. *Lyme disease. Mon parcours pour retrouver la santé.* Vergèze, Thierry Souccar Éditions, 2012.

Benarrosh S. *À la recherche de ma santé perdue.* Paris, Editions du Moment, 2015.

Berche P. *Une histoire des microbes.* Paris, John Libbey Eurotext, 2007.

Carroll MC. *Lab 257. Caution: The disturbing story of the Government's secret germ laboratory.* New York, HarperCollins Publishers, 2004.

CMIT (Collège des Universitaires de Maladies Infectieuses et Tropicales). *E Pilly: Infectious and tropical diseases 2016.* 25th edition, Paris, Alinéa Plus, 2016.

Foucaut M. *Lyme disease: The silent epidemic. A fight for our lives.* Paris, Josette Lyon, 2015.

Freney J, Renaud F. *La Guerre des microbes de l'Antiquité au 11 Septembre 2001.* Paris, Éditions Eska, 2009.

Horowitz R. *Why can't I get better? Solving the mystery of Lyme & chronic disease.* New York, St Martin's Press, 2013. French translation: *Soigner Lyme & les maladies chroniques inexpliquées.* Vergèze, Thierry Souccar Éditions, 2014.

Institute of Medicine (US) Committee on Quality of Health Care in America. *Crossing the quality chasm: a new health system for the 21st century.* Washington DC, National Academies Press, 2001.

Jadin C. *Une maladie appelée fatigue.* Brussels, Artcadia Éditions, 2002.

Kupiec J-J, Sonigo P. *Ni Dieu ni gène. Pour une autre théorie de l'hérédité.* Paris, Seuil, 2000.

Kraaijeveld H. *Shifting the Lyme paradigm. The characters' guide on a hero's journey.* Utrecht, Stili Novi Publishing, 2014 (accessible online: http://huib.me/en/work/ shifting-the-lyme-paradigm).

Le Saux E. *Face à Lyme. Journal d'un naufrage.* Paris, Michalon Éditeur, 2015.

Leibowitch J. *Pour en finir avec le sida.* Paris, Plon, 2011.
Lenglet R, Perrin C. *L'affaire de la maladie de Lyme. Une enquête.* Arles, Actes Sud, 2016.
Liegner KB. *In the crucible of chronic Lyme disease.* Bloomington, Indiana, Xlibris, 2015.
Luché-Thayer J, Ahern H, DellaSala D et al. *Updating ICD11 borreliosies diagnostic codes.* Scotts Valley, California, CreateSpace Independent Publishing Platform, 2017.
Luché-Thayer J, Ahern H, Bransfield R, et al. *The situation of human rights defenders of Lyme and relapsing fever borreliosis. The Ad Hoc Committee for Health Equity in ICD11 Borreliosis Codes.* Scotts Valley, California, CreateSpace Independent Publishing Platform, 2018.
Luché-Thayer J, Skidmore D. *$lyme: How medical codes mortally wound corruption and scientific fraud.* Scotts Valley, California, CreateSpace Independent Publishing Platform, 2018.
Margulis L, Sagan D. *Microcosmos. Four billion years of evolution from our microbial ancestors.* New York, Simon & Schuster, Inc. 1986; French translation: *L'Univers bactériel. Les nouveaux rapports de l'homme et de la nature.* Paris, Albin Michel, 1989.
Nicolle C. *Destin des maladies infectieuses.* Paris, Librairie Félix Alcan, 1933; reprinted by the Association des Anciens Élèves de l'Institut Pasteur, Paris, France Lafayette edition, 1993.
Payer L. *Medicine and culture.* New York, Henry Holt and Company LLC, 1988, 1996.
Raoult D. Epidémies : vrais dangers et fausses alertes. Michel Lafon, Neuilly sur Seine. 2020
Raxlen B, Cashel A. *Lyme disease – medical myopia and the hidden global pandemic: A guide to navigating the labyrinth of diagnosis and treatment.* London, Hammersmith Health Books, 2019.
Pfeiffer MB. *Lyme. The first epidemic of climate change.* Washington, Island Press, 2018.
Piel F. *J'ai peur d'oublier.* Paris, Michel Lafon, 2009.
Schaller V. *Lyme disease. L'épidémie qu'on vous cache.* Vergèze, Thierry Souccar Éditions, 2015.
Sackett D, Straus S, Richardson W, et al. *Evidence-based medicine: how to practise and teach EBM.* Edinburgh, Churchill Livingstone, 2000.

Weblinks

Agency for Healthcare Research and Quality.
Recommendations of ILADS (International Lyme and Associated Diseases Society). Evidence assessments and guideline recommendations in Lyme disease: the clinical management of known tick bites, erythema migrans rashes and persistent disease: www.guideline.gov/content. aspx?id=49320

Centers for Disease Control and Prevention (CDC), National notifiable diseases surveillance system (NNdSS). Lyme disease (Borrelia burgdorferi) 2011 case definition: wwwn.cdc.gov/nndss/conditions/lyme-disease/case-definition/2011/

Centers for Disease Control and Prevention. CDC provides estimates of Americans diagnosed with Lyme disease each year: www.cdc.gov/media/releases/2013/ p0819-lyme-disease.html

European Concerted Action on Lyme Borreliosis (EUCALB), diagnosis. Serology: minimum standards: http://meduni09.edis.at/eucalb/cms_15/index.php?option=com_content&view=article&id=39:serology-minimum-standards&catid=62: diagnosis-serology&Itemid=70.
Note: the EUCALB website disappeared in 2017.

Haut Conseil de la santé publique. Mieux connaître la borréliose de Lyme pour mieux la prévenir, 29 janvier 2010: www.hcsp.fr/Explore.cgi/avisrapports- domaine?clefr=138

Haut Conseil de la santé publique. Borréliose de Lyme. état des connaissances, 28 mars 2014: www.hcsp.fr/Explore.cgi/avisrapportsdomaine?clefr=465

Haut Conseil de la santé publique. Borréliose de Lyme. modes de transmission, 19 février 2016: www.hcsp.fr/Explore.cgi/avisrapportsdomaine?clefr=564

European Centre for Disease prevention and Control. April 2016. A systematic literature review on the diagnostic accuracy of serological tests for Lyme borreliosis: https://ecdc.europa.eu/sites/portal/files/media/en/publications/Publications/lyme-borreliosis-diagnostic-accuracy-serological-tests-systematic-review.pdf

US Department of Health and Human Services. 2018. Tick borne diseases working group reports: www.hhs.gov/ash/advisory-committees/tickbornedisease/reports

US Department of Health and Human Services. 2018
Tick-Borne Disease Working Group 2018 Report to Congress: www.hhs.gov/sites/default/files/tbdwg-report-to-congress-2018.pdf?fbclid=IwAR1u5BTMGMUMCIdMOfudGAqChW1psJL421l76FXWWn4u-YYh2edmRR0LHyw

Haute Autorité de Santé (HAS). 2018.
French recommendations of good clinical practice: Lyme disease and other tick-borne diseases (in French): www.has-sante.fr/portail/upload/docs/application/pdf/2018-06/reco266_rbp_borreliose_de_lyme_cd_2018_06_13__recommandations.pdf

Index

Index

Also from Hammersmith Health Books

Rethinking Pain

– How to live with chronic pain

By Dr Helena Miranda

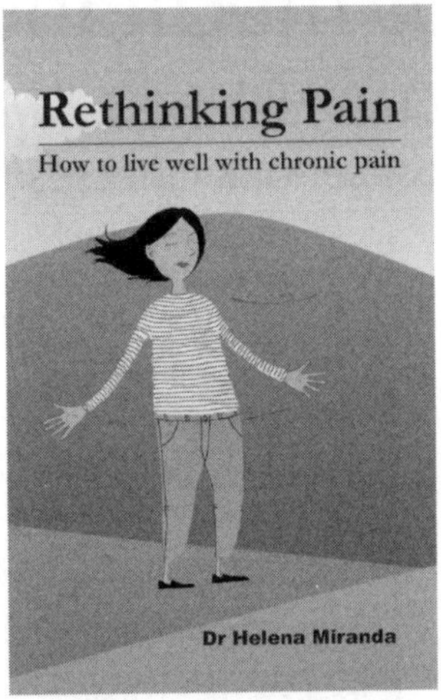

While medicines may help with acute pain they have little impact on long-term chronic pain other than dependency and the need for ever increasing doses. But there are many tried-and-tested alternatives for chronic pain that do not involve drugs, are non-addictive and even beneficial in other ways. Occupational physician and chronic pain sufferer, Dr Miranda, has developed this practical and empathetic guide to a revolutionary approach to living well with chronic pain, based on the fundamental principles that: all pain experienced is real; all pain is experienced in the brain; all pain is unique to the sufferer; the key to overcoming pain is not to strive to be pain-free but to minimise the *experience*.

Also from Hammersmith Health Books

Curing the Incurable: Beyond the limits of medicine

– How those who have recovered from today's most serious illnesses succeeded

By Dr Jerry Thompson

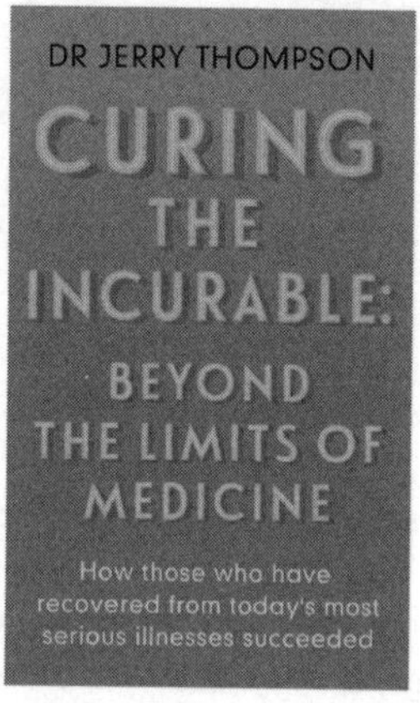

Dr Jerry Thompson draws on an immense range of case histories and research studies to show how what we eat, the toxic load we carry, the environmental electromagnetic fields we live in, and our beliefs and attitudes to health and illness can change the course of disease. The result is a practical guide to what we can learn from 'survivors' about how to improve our chances of good health and recovery.

Also from Hammersmith Health Books

Could it be Insulin Resistance?

By Hanna Purdy

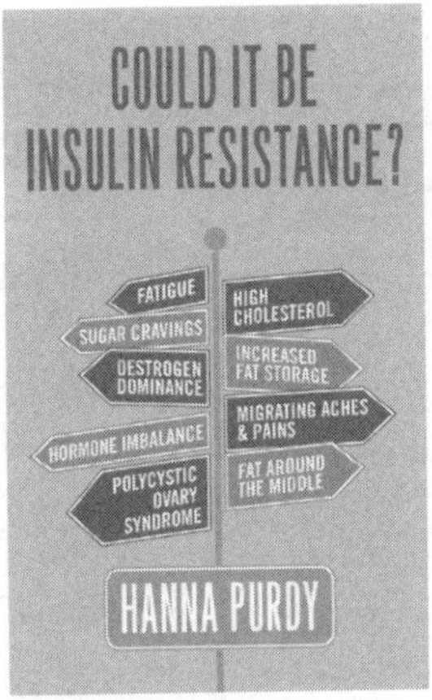

Nurse Practitioner Hanna Purdy shares her long experience in Public Health Nursing, as well as with improving her own family's health, to present this practical, evidence-based guide to what 'insulin resistance' means, what causes it and what to do about it, including how to start a ketogenic/low-carb diet, with the emphasis on the quality of food eaten and the impact good food can have on the body and mind. As she shows, insulin resistance is caused by chronic, sub-clinical inflammation and lies behind many common chronic illnesses that are now reaching epidemic levels even in children.

Also from Hammersmith Health Books

The Infection Game

Life is an arms race

By Dr Sarah Myhill and Craig Robinson

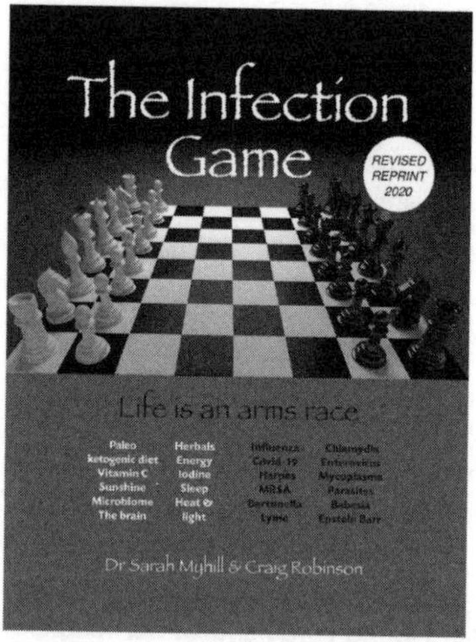

The Infection Game shows us how we can maximise our defences and martial our weapons, cheaply and effectively, so that we are ready to defeat the infectious organisms we encounter every day and in epidemic situations.

Also from Hammersmith Health Books

The Infection Game Supplement

By Dr Sarah Myhill and Craig Robinson

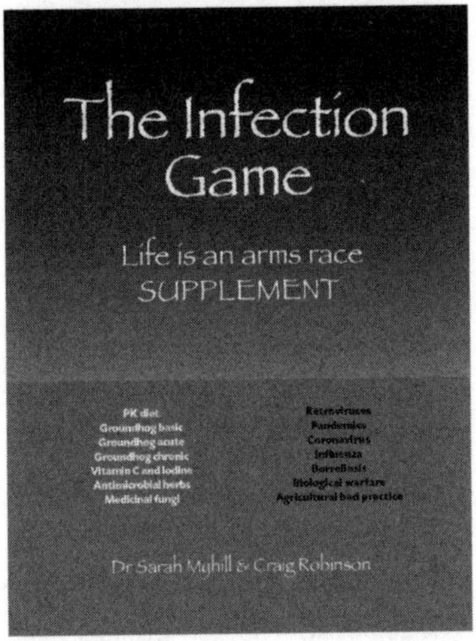

Three additional, essential chapters for readers of The Infection Game on Retroviruses, Pandemics and the Rise of new infective organisms.
(Available as an ebook only)

Also from Hammersmith Health Books

Lyme Disease

Medical myopia and the hidden global pandemic

Dr Bernard Raxlen and Allie Cashel

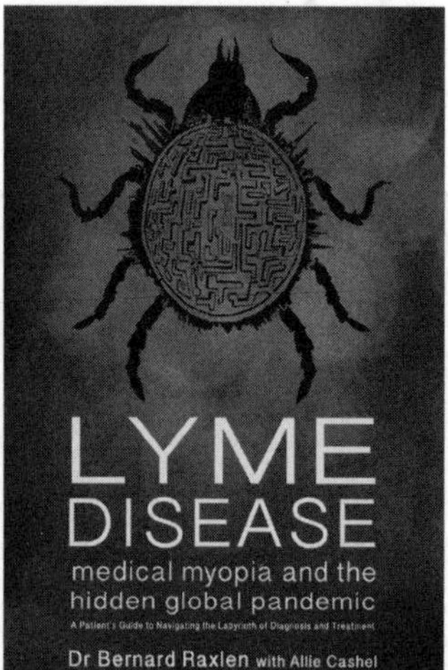

Based on years of diagnosing and treating this growing problem in NY City, Dr Raxlen, together with 'expert patient' Allie Cashel and a team of international contributors, provides a road map for individuals who suspect they have been infected and are lost in the 'medical maze' of Lyme and other tick-borne diseases, searching for a diagnosis and appropriate treatment. By highlighting the difficulties sufferers face, Raxlen et al aim to increase understanding of the Lyme epidemic worldwide and how sufferers can obtain reliable and effective diagnosis and treatment.